Clinical Methods i

Obstetrics and Gyr

Clinical Methods in Obstetrics and Gynecology

Second Edition

PN Nobis MBBS MD (OBG)
Senior Consultant
Department of Obstetrics and Gynecology
International Hospital
Guwahati, Assam, India
Former Professor and Head
Department of Obstetrics and Gynecology
Silchar Medical College
Silchar, Assam, India

Foreword
Bharati Barooah

JAYPEE

JAYPEE BROTHERS MEDICAL PUBLISHERS (P) LTD
New Delhi • London • Philadelphia • Panama

Jaypee Brothers Medical Publishers (P) Ltd

Headquarters
Jaypee Brothers Medical Publishers (P) Ltd
4838/24, Ansari Road, Daryaganj
New Delhi 110 002, India
Phone: +91-11-43574357
Fax: +91-11-43574314
Email: jaypee@jaypeebrothers.com

Overseas Offices

J.P. Medical Ltd
83 Victoria Street, London
SW1H 0HW (UK)
Phone: +44-2031708910
Fax: +02-03-0086180
Email: info@jpmedpub.com

Jaypee-Highlights Medical Publishers Inc
City of Knowledge, Bld. 237, Clayton
Panama City, Panama
Phone: + 507-301-0496
Fax: + 507-301-0499
Email: cservice@jphmedical.com

Jaypee Medical Inc
The Bourse
111 South Independence Mall East
Suite 835, Philadelphia, PA 19106, USA
Phone: + 267-519-9789
Email: joe.rusko@jaypeebrothers.com

Jaypee Brothers Medical Publishers (P) Ltd
17/1-B Babar Road, Block-B, Shaymali
Mohammadpur, Dhaka-1207
Bangladesh
Mobile: +08801912003485
Email: jaypeedhaka@gmail.com

Jaypee Brothers Medical Publishers (P) Ltd
Shorakhute, Kathmandu
Nepal
Phone: +00977-9841528578
Email: jaypee.nepal@gmail.com

Website: www.jaypeebrothers.com
Website: www.jaypeedigital.com

Inquiries for bulk sales may be solicited at: jaypee@jaypeebrothers.com

Clinical Methods in Obstetrics and Gynecology

First Edition: 1997

Second Edition: **2014**

ISBN: 978-81-8448-989-7

Printed at: S.Narayan & Sons

Foreword

I have the pleasure of going through the book entitled *Clinical Methods in Obstetrics and Gynecology* authored by Dr PN Nobis. The book is a comprehensive and updated textbook for both undergraduate and postgraduate students of obstetrics and gynecology. Moreover, the author has discussed some practical problems faced by doctors in history taking and clinical examination of pregnant women in our society where ignorance, taboos and superstitions are prevalent. Therefore, the book is very informative and useful guide for the doctors dealing with obstetric cases, particularly in rural areas.

The detection and management of high-risk pregnancies, including their early referral to well-equipped hospitals whenever necessary, are very important steps to reduce the maternal and perinatal mortality and morbidity rates. This book contains a chapter on "High-Risk Pregnancy" that would be of immense help for the students as well as the practicing doctors.

I hope the book will receive due recognition and appreciation.

Bharati Barooah MBBS FRCOG (London)
Professor
Department of Obstetrics and Gynecology
Guwahati Medical College
Guwahati, Assam, India

Preface to the Second Edition

This is the second edition of the previous book titled "Clinical Methods in Obstetrics". In this edition gynecological portion is added and the name of the book is changed to *Clinical Methods in Obstetrics and Gynecology*. Few more chapters of obstetrics are added and the previous chapters are reviewed and elaborated. Looking back to the anatomy and physiology classes, an attempt is made to recapitulate the basics of female genital organs. Theoretical part of every chapter is reviewed before beginning the clinical examination, necessary investigations, and their interpretation.

Several of my past students and colleagues have rendered their valuable help in preparing the book. I am really indebted to them. I am very grateful to Dr Jayanti Chanda Das, Dr Karabi Patowary and Dr Kamal Kathar, for their excellent photography. I am also thankful to Dr Debjani Roy Chaudhury and Dr Iheule N Khiangte, for helping me in many ways while compiling the book. It is Latika and Nipak of Baruah Photostat, Bhangagarh and Mr PP Nath, who should be credited for computer typing of the whole manuscript. I am specially grateful to my wife Mrs Aruna Nobis, for her constant encouragement and necessary help and to my two kids Suman and Pahi, for their help in computer works at home.

Finally, it is Shri Jitendar P Vij (Group Chairman), Mr Ankit Vij (Managing Director) and Mr Tarun Duneja (Director-Publishing) of M/s Jaypee Brothers Medical Publishers (P) Ltd, New Delhi, India, who came forward to publish the book. I am happy to express my gratefulness to them.

My work will be rewarded provided the students, for whom it is prepared, are benefited.

PN Nobis

Preface to the Second Edition

Preface to the First Edition

The purpose of this book is to help the new comers who have just been introduced to the subject—obstetrics. There are several excellent textbooks on obstetrics. In all those books, methods of clinical examination and interpretation of the findings are scattered throughout. Here an attempt is made to reproduce them together in a simple manner. The need of such a book was felt while taking bedside clinics for the junior students for several years and I was prompted to prepare this. The actual work was started much earlier, but it took a long time to bring the book out. During this time, I am lucky to get help and encouragement from many of my friends and colleagues. I am specially indebted to Dr (Ms) Bharati Barooah, FRCOG, for patiently going through the manuscript and for her valuable suggestions and encouragement. She was very kind to write the foreword of the book. Again, my pediatrician friend Dr CS Das, MD, Professor, Department of Pediatrics, Silchar Medical College, Assam, India, rendered valuable help in the pediatric section. I am very much grateful to him. I am also grateful to Dr (Mrs) Saswati Sanyal Chaudhury, MD, Assistant Professor, Department of Obstetrics and Gynecology, Guwahati Medical College, Assam, India, for her valuable suggestions and constant encouragement. My thanks are due to Mr Apurba Gogoi and Mr Atanu Chaudhury, for the illustrations and to Mr B Saikia, for typing the manuscript. It gives me pleasure to offer my heartiest thanks to my elder brother Sri CD Nobis and to Sri DK Saikia, for their much needed help. My friend Dr NK Barua of National Printers, Guwahati, needs special mention, for taking the responsibility to bring out the book to light.

At last, it is my sincere hope that the book will be of some help to them for whom it is meant—my junior students.

PN Nobis

Contents

chapter

1

Female Genital Organs

The reproductive system of woman is described in two parts – external reproductive organ and internal reproductive organ.

❐ EXTERNAL REPRODUCTIVE ORGANS

The part of female reproductive organs that can be seen from outside is external reproductive organ. The main parts are: mons veneris or mons pubis – the swollen fat filled area covering the pubic symphysis is mons veneris. It is covered by luxuriant growth of black curly hair.

Labia Majora

Labia majora extends downwards and backwards from the mons pubis. Posteriorly the two labia majora of either side joint in the midline together to form the posterior commissure. In children and in nulliparous women they cover the underlying parts. These are two skin folds filled with fat.

Labia Minora

Labia minora are two folds of tissue inside the labia majora. They meet at the upper end of vulva and posteriorly meet at the middle to form fourchet. In nulliparous women, they are covered by the labia majora.

Clitoris

Clitoris is situated in the midline just above the labia minora. It is a small erectile body homologous of the penis. Like the penis it consists of a glans, a body and two crura. It is very sensitive.

Vestibule

The area enclosed by the labia minora is vestibule. It extends from the clitoris anteriorly to the fourchet posteriorly. It is perforated by the urethra and vagina. Besides these there are openings of two skene's ducts and openings of the Bartholin's glands.

Urethral Meatus

Urethra opens at the urethral meatus in the midline of the vestibule. It is situated above the vaginal opening. The orifice appears as a vertical slit.

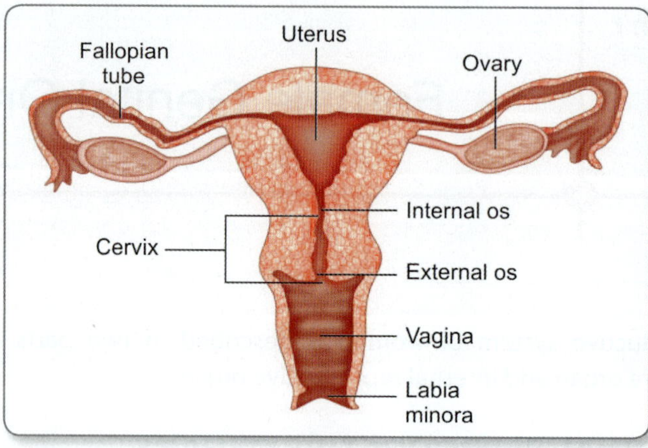

Fig. 1: Uterus with tubes and ovaries

❐ VAGINAL OPENING

Vaginal opening is situated at the lower part of the vestibule. Its size and shape is variable. In virgin it is almost closed by hymen, a membrane. The hymen may be perforated at places. During the first coitus the hymen ruptures. After child birth the remnants of hymen form cicatrized nodules called myrtiform caruncles (caruncle myrtiformes).

Vagina

Vagina is a musculomembranous tube, interposed between the urinary bladder and rectum. It extends from vulva to the cervix of the uterus. In the upper part vagina is blind and the lower portion of the cervix projects into it. The blind end is called vault. The vault is divided into anterior, posterior and lateral fornices. Posteriorly vagina is attached to the cervix at a higher level than on the anterior, so the posterior fornix is deeper than the anterior one. Length of vagina varies, anteriorly it is about 6–8 cm and posteriorly is about 7–10 cm. The vaginal canal is usually H-shaped.

Inside the vaginal canal there are few longitudinal ridges and there are numerous transverse ridges or rugae.

The mucosa of the vagina is lined by stratified squamous epithelium. Next to the epithelial layer is the fibromuscular layer. This smooth muscle layer is composed of inner circular layer and outer longitudinal layer. Vagina is devoid of glands. The superficial mucosal cells contain glycogen. Examination of the superficial mucosal cells give indication of effect of ovarian hormonal pattern. This is of clinical importance. Vagina is kept moist by secretion from uterus. Glycogen of the mucosal cells are broken down by lactobacilli forming lactic acid that keeps the vagina acidic. In adult women vaginal pH is between 4.0 and 5.0.

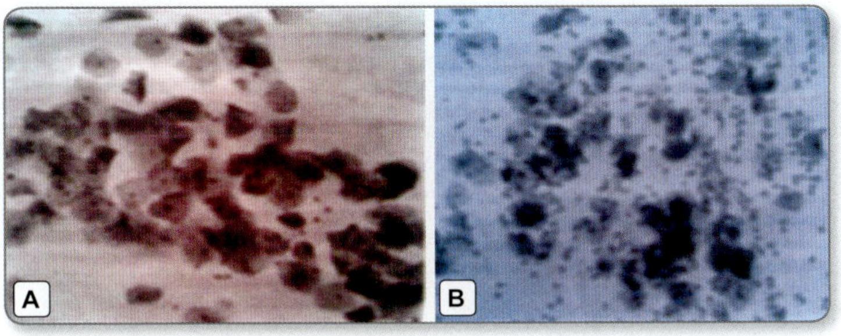

Fig. 2: Vaginal smear during. (A) proliferative phase shows large cells with pyknotic nuclei; (B) during secretory phase, many cells are rolled edge and with large numbers of leukocytes

The Perineum

The area between the posterior fourchette and the anus is perineum. Perineum is made up of superficial perineal muscles and external anal sphincter. The median raphe of levator ani reinforced by these muscles form the perineal body.

Blood supply and nerve supply

Uterus: The uterus is a pear-shaped muscular organ. Usually the length of the uterus is 7.5 cm, breath is 5 cm and 2.5 cm thick. In non-pregnant state uterus is situated inside the pelvic cavity. The urinary bladder is situated anteriorly and the rectum posteriorly. The upper part is wide narrowing gradually downwards. The triangular upper part is body and cylindrical lower portion is cervix. The two fallopian tubes enter the uterus at its two upper corners laterally. The part of the uterus above the attachment of the fallopian tubes is called the fundus of the uterus. A small segment between the body and the cervix is known as isthmus.

The cavity of the uterus is triangular in shape. As the walls are thick the cavity is small. The anterior and the posterior walls are almost in contact with each other. The opening in the upper part of the cervix is called internal os and the opening at the lower end is external os.

The cervix is just bellow the isthmus. The part of the cervix above the attachment of vagina is supravaginal portion and the part below is portio vaginalis. Cervix is composed of connective tissue, elastic tissue and few smooth muscle fibers. The mucosa of cervix, though continuous with endometrium, has different characteristics. It is composed of a single layer of columnar epithelium. There are numerous cervical glands, which extend from the mucosa to deep into the underlying connective tissue. The outer surface of the portio vaginalis is covered with squamous epithelium. This layer of squamous epithelium and the columnar epithelium of the cervical canal meet near the external os at the squamocolumnar junction.

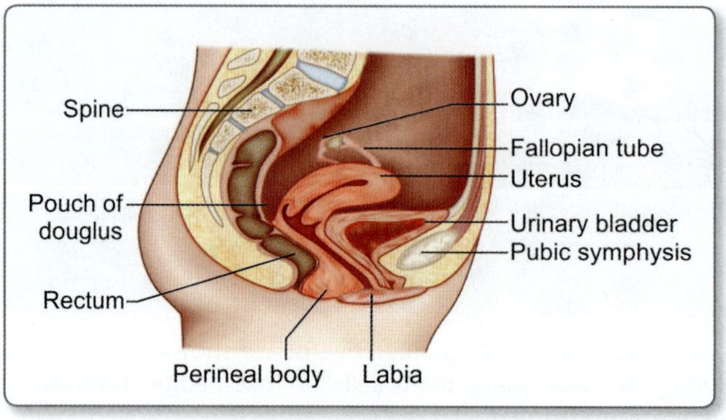

Fig. 3: Relation of uterus with urinary bladder and rectum

The wall of the body of the uterus is made up of three layers – serosal, muscular and mucous membrane. The serosal layer is the peritoneal covering. The muscular layer is known as myometrium. It is composed of bundle of smooth muscle united by connective tissue. The mucosal layers covering the uterine cavity is endometrium. It is thin, pink and velvety layer. The endometrium undergoes continuous changes during menstrual cycle. It is composed of a single layer of surface epithelium, glands and stroma. Stroma is richly supplied with blood vessels.

Blood Supply

The uterine and the ovarian arteries supply the uterus. Uterine artery is a branch of internal iliac artery, and the ovarian artery comes directly from the abdominal aorta. Arising from the internal iliac artery the uterine artery descends downwards and medially to enter into the base of the broad ligament. There it crosses over the ureter. Near the cervix it divides into two parts. The smaller cervicovaginal branch supplies the lower part of the cervix and the upper part of the vagina. The bigger branch turns upwards and runs upwards as a convoluted vessel along the lateral margin of the uterus. While running upwards it gives numerous branches that enters into the substance of the uterus. At the upper end the ovarian branch anastomose with ovarian artery. Another branch supply the tube and the third one supply the fundus of the uterus.

On either side the arcuate veins unite to form the uterine vein. The uterine veins accompany the uterine arteries and drain into the internal iliac veins.

Ligaments of the Uterus

The uterus is held in position by some thick bands of fibrous tissue called ligaments. These fibrous tissues are continuous with connective tissue of the pelvis. Extending from the lateral border of the uterus are broad ligaments, round ligament and cardinal ligaments or Mackenrodt's ligament.

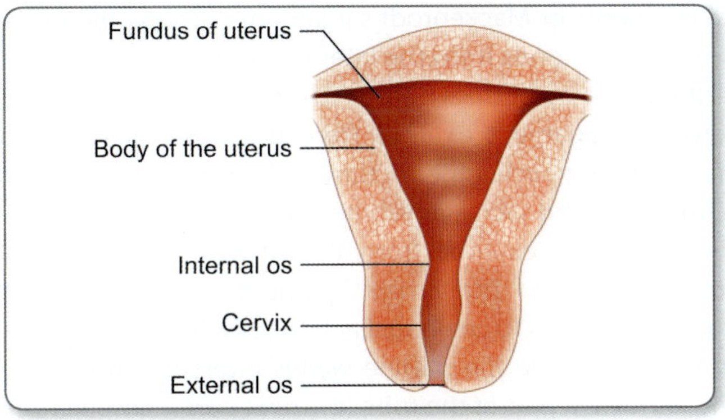

Fig. 4: Different parts of uterus

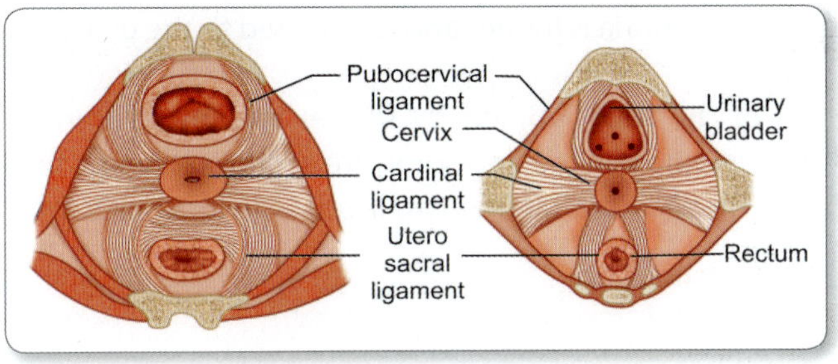

Fig. 5: Ligaments of uterus

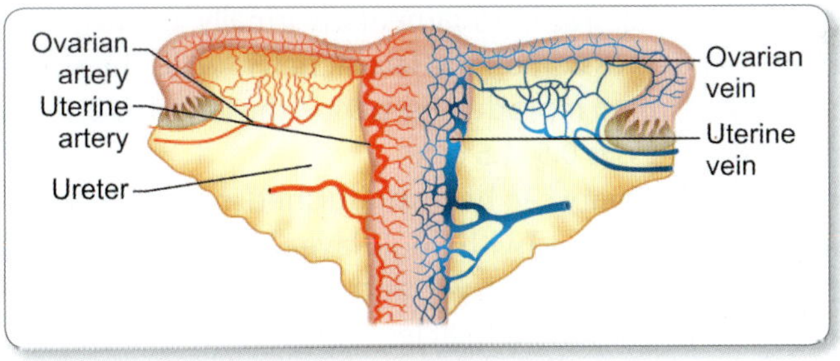

Fig. 6: Blood supply of uterus

The broad ligament consists of two layers of periotineum extending from the lateral margin of the uterus to the lateral pelvic wall. It envelops various structures. Inner two-thirds covers the fallopian tube and is known as mesosalpinx. The free lateral one-third is known as infundibulopelvic ligaments. It contains the ovarian vessels.

The round ligaments extend from the upper lateral corner of the uterus. It arises from anterior and below the origin of the fallopian tubes. It runs downwards and laterally to enter the inguinal canal, passing through the canal terminate in the labia majus.

Cardinal ligaments or Mackenrodt's ligaments occupy the lower margin of broad ligaments. It extends from the lateral margin of the cervix to the lateral pelvic wall. It is made up of thick fibrous tissue.

The uterosacral ligament extends from the posterolateral aspect of the supravaginal cervix, encircles the rectum and inserts into the fascia covering the second and the third sacral vertebrae. It is covered by peritoneum.

The fallopian tubes extends from the uterine cervix. It is covered by peritoneum. This part of the broad ligament is called mesosalpinx. The fallopian tubes are about 10 cm long. Each tube is divided into four parts – the part which remains inside the uterine wall is interstitial portion, next to it is isthmus, the narrowest part of the tube, the next part is ampulla which is wider than isthmus. The last part is infundibulum or the fimbriated end. It is funnel-shaped and opens in the peritoneal cavity. It has some finger-like processes called fimbria. One fimbria is longer and is attached to the ovary. This is fimbria ovarica.

The lumen of the tube is lined by single layer of columnar epithelium. Some of these cells are ciliated and some are secretory. Below this layer is the muscular layer. The musculature has two layers – an inner circular and an outer longitudinal layer.

The Ovaries

On either side of the uterus there are two ovaries. Ovaries are suspended from the broad ligament by mesovarium and are attached to the posterolateral aspects of the uterus with ovarian ligaments. Normally, the ovaries are situated at ovarian fossa—a depression on the lateral pelvic wall. The size of the ovary varies considerably. During reproductive period the length is 2.5–5 cm, breadth is 1.5–3 cm and thickness is 0.5–1.5 cm.

The structure of the ovary can be distinguished into two parts – cortex and medulla. The surface is covered with single layer of epithelium, called germinal epithelium. Cortex is the outer layer and its thickness varies according to age. In this layer, the primordial follicles and Graafian follicles are scattered. During each menstrual cycle few primordial follicles develop and only one matures and develops into a Graafian follicle and ruptures during ovulation

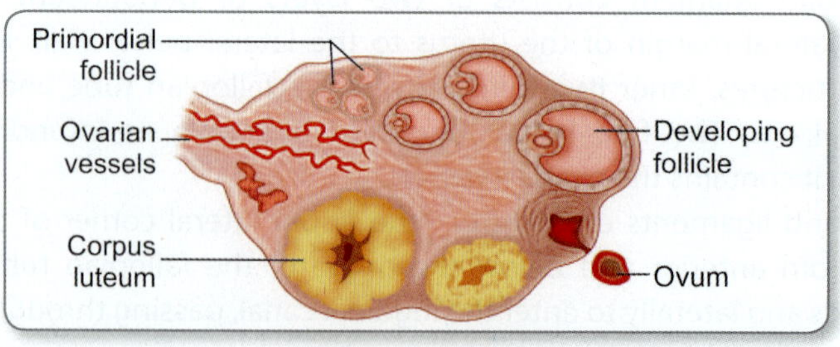

Fig. 7: Ovary

to liberate the ovum. After ovulation it forms corpus luteum. Later on the follicle becomes fibrous and whitish in color. This is called tunica albuginea. The medulla is composed of loose connective tissue. Medulla contains blood vessels and few smooth muscle fibers.

The functions of ovaries are to secret ovarian steroids—oestrogen and progestogens and production of ovum. The ovum comes out of ovary during the ovulation.

Ovaries are supplied by the ovarian arteries, branch of the abdominal aorta. The accompanying veins drain impure blood to the inferior vena cava.

❐ EMBRYOLOGICAL DEVELOPMENT

Uterus and Fallopian Tubes

The uterus and the fallopian tubes develop from the Müllerian ducts. Müllerian ducts appear at the upper part of the urogenital ridge by 5th week of intrauterine life. From the upper part of the Müllerian ducts develop the fallopian tubes. The lower parts of the tubes of both sides fuse in the midline and later on the intervening walls disappear to form the uterus and vagina below.

The Ovaries

The ovaries develop from the genital ridge, an area in the urogenital ridge medial to the area wherefrom the Müllerian ducts originate. Germ cells migrate to this area from an area in the coelomic epithelium. The germ cells appear there by about 3rd week of intrauterine life and migrate to the genital ridge by fifth week. The development of ovum continues till term.

Breast

In female, breasts are secondary sex organ. During puberty size of the breast increases due to effects of hormones. It is composed of glands and fatty tissues.

It is a circular organ rising gradually towards the center. At the middle the skin is raised. It is called nipple. Surrounding the nipple is a circular brown area, the areola. In the areola there are some raised areas. These are sebaceous glands beneath the skin. About 15–20 ducts open at the tip of the nipple.

The breast is a gland, it is composed of several small lobules. These are separated by connective tissue. Each lobule is again constituted by several glandular sac. Tubules of several lobules join together to form a lactiferous sinus. Then again take the shape of a duct and opens at the tip of the nipple. The lobules draining in one lactiferous duct form a lobe.

Blood Supply of Pelvis

Pelvis is richly supplied with blood vessels. These vessels not only supplies the genital organs but also supply the lower urinary tract, gastrointestinal tract, pelvic floor and perineum. The major vessels supplying the pelvis are –

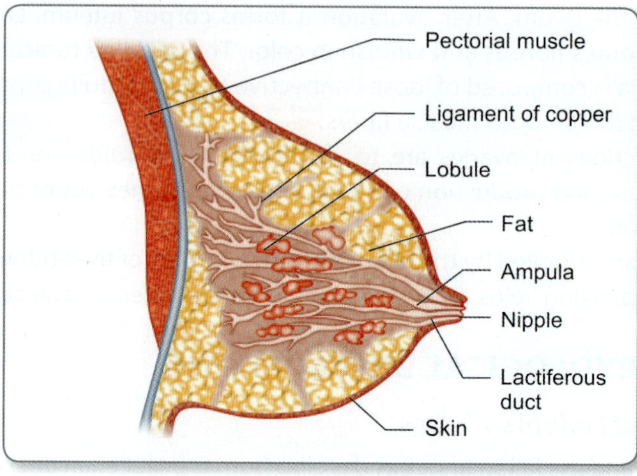

Fig. 8: Structure of human breast

internal iliac artery and ovarian artery. There is extensive collateral connections between different vessels supplying the pelvis.

Internal Iliac Artery

The abdominal aorta bifurcates at the level of fifth lumber vertebra, into two common iliac arteries. Running downwards and outwards the common iliac artery bifurcate into external and internal iliac arteries. The external iliac artery runs downwards and outwards and passing below the inguinal ligament becomes femoral artery. Its main branches are inferior epigastric and deep circumflex arteries.

The internal iliac artery descends into the pelvis and at the level of the greater sciatic foramen divides into anterior and posterior divisions. The posterior division passes through the foramen and supplies the muscles of the buttock. The anterior division supplies the pelvic organs. Its branches are: superior vesical, inferior vesical, middle rectal, uterine, vaginal and obturator. The terminal branches are internal pudendal and inferior gluteal arteries.

Uterine Artery

The uterine artery arises from the internal iliac artery directly or with the superior vesical artery. Running inwards at the base of the broad ligament crosses the ureter anteriorly and reaches the uterus at the level of the internal os. At this level it divides into two, one descending branch to supply the cervix and vagina. The main branch runs upwards along the lateral border of the uterus. It is tortuous and gives off branches to supply the uterus at all levels and at last anastomose with the ovarian artery. The branches from the main artery divides into anterior and posterior arcuate arteries which run circumferencially

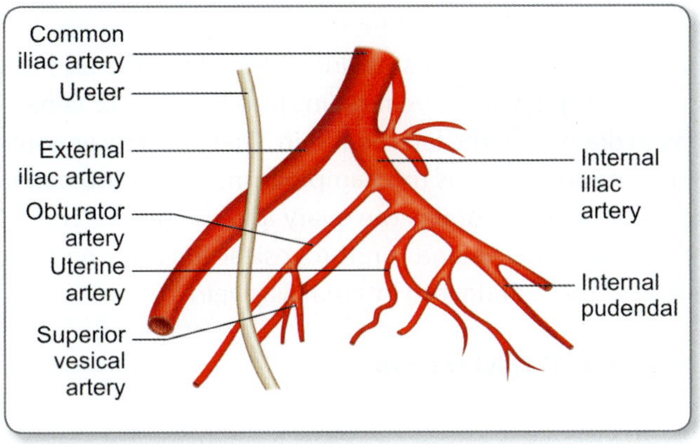

Fig. 9: Arterial supply of pelvis

in the myometrium and anastomose with those from the opposite side. The arcuate arteries give off radial arteries which end as basal arteries and supply the endometrium. Arcuate and radial arteries are also coiled.

Vaginal Artery

The vaginal artery usually arises directly from the internal iliac artery and running forwards and inwards in the lower part of the broad ligament reaches the lateral fornix of vagina. In the vaginal fornix it anastomoses with branches of cervical artery. It supplies the upper vagina. The lower vagina is supplied by the middle and inferior rectal arteries and by branches of the internal pudendal artery.

Internal Pudendal Artery

The internal pudendal artery is the terminal branch of the internal iliac artery. It passes out of the pelvis through the greater sciatic notch. It gives branches to supply the labia, vagina, vestibule, perineum and perineal muscles. It ends as the dorsal artery to clitoris.

Ovarian Artery

The ovarian artery is a branch of abdominal aorta. It runs retroperitonealy downwards and laterally. At the level of the brim of the pelvis it crosses the ureter and then enters the infundibulopelvic ligament. It divides into two branches. The main one reaches the ovary through the mesovarian. The other branch or the main trunk itself runs towards the cornu of the uterus and anastomose with the uterine artery. In the mesosalpinx vessels supply the round ligament and the fallopian tube from the vascular arch formed by the anastomosis of the ovarian and uterine arteries.

Veins

The veins accompany the arteries having the same name and drain into the internal iliac vein. Right ovarian vein drains into the inferior venacava and the left ovarian vein drains into the left renal vein. There are few venous plexuses in the pelvis. The important one is the pampiniform plexus situated in the upper part of broad ligament and drains the ovary and the uterus. The other venous plexuses are around the vagina, urethrovesical junction and the anorectal junction and all of them drain into internal iliac vein.

❐ LYMPHATIC DRAINAGE

Vulva

Lymphatics of vulva pass towards the mons pubis to enter into the medial group of superficial inguinal lymph nodes, then to the deep inguinal group. From deep inguinal group of glands lymphatics drain into the external iliac lymph nodes. Gland of Cloquet is situated beneath the inner end of the inguinal ligament. Lymphatics from clitoris directly drains into this gland when present. Lymphatics from the deeper tissues drain into the internal iliac nodes.

Vagina

Lymphatics from lower vagina accompany the lymphatics of vulva and drain into the inguinal and femoral nodes. From upper part lymphatics accompany those from cervix.

Cervix

Lymphatics from cervix drain into the obturator, external and internal iliac and sacral nodes. From cervix these lymphatics pass through the uterosacral ligaments to these glands. External and internal iliac nodes ultimately drain into the para-aortic lymph glands.

Body of the Uterus

Upper part of the body of the uterus including the fundus are drained by lymphatics accompanying the ovarian vessels. Some lymphatics pass through the round ligament to the superficial inguinal nodes. The lower part has same lymphatic connection as in cervix.

Ovary and fallopian tube are drained by lymphatics accompanying the ovarian vessels and communicate with the aortic nodes. Some vessels from the tube run along with the lymphatics from fundus of the uterus.

Nerve Supply

The pudendal nerve is the main somatic supply of the pelvic organs. It has both motor and sensory fibers derived from the S2, S3 and S4 roots of the sacral plexus.

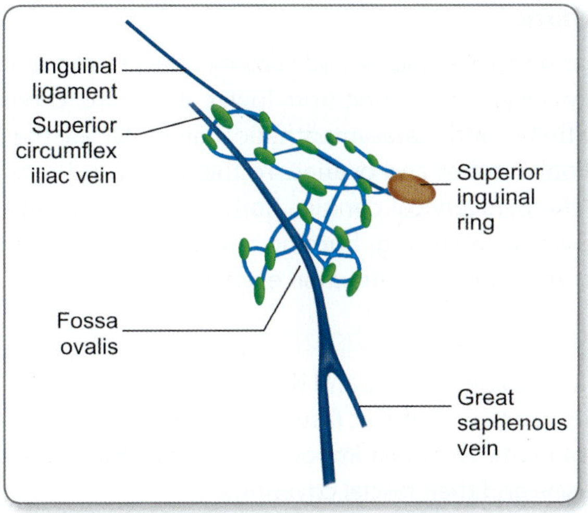

Fig. 10: Inguinal lymph nodes

The motor fibers supply the voluntary muscles, vaginal sphincter, compressor urethrae, levator ani and external anal sphincter. The sensory fibers supply the skin of vulva, clitoris, external urethral meatus, lower vagina and perineum.

The pudendal nerve leaves the pelvis through the greater sciatic notch, circles around the ischial spine and re-enters the pelvis through the lesser sciatic notch. Ischial spine is an important landmark to inject local anesthetic solution for pudendal block.

Skin of the mons pubis and anterior part of vulva is also supplied by ilioinguinal nerve and the genital branch of the genitofemoral nerve (L1 and L2 roots).

Autonomic Nerves

Autonomic nervous system regulates the activities of all the internal reproductive organs including upper vagina, urinary system, rectum and colon. These nerves carry both motor and sensory fibers. Nerves to and from the genital organs pass through some plexuses.

Sympathetic

Sympathetic motor nerves arise from the T5 and T6 segments and sensory nerves arise from the T10 to L1 segments. These nerve go downwards from the coeliac plexus to the presacral plexus or the superior hypogastric plexus, situated over the bifurcation of the aorta and sacral promontory. Therefrom two hypogastric nerves run downwards and outwards, one on each side to join the inferior hypogastric plexus or the pelvic plexus. The pelvic plexus extends forwards beneath the uterosacral and broad ligaments.

Parasympathetic

Pelvic plexus also receives motor and sensory fibers from S2, S3 and S4 nerve roots, probably carrying sensation from lower uterus and cervix. Pelvic plexus supply sympathetic and parasympathetic nerves to all the pelvic organs except the fallopian tubes and ovaries. To the uterus and cervix these nerves pass through the paracervical ganglia. Body of the uterus and the cervix are relatively insensitive to cutting, burning, etc. Resection of all uterine nerves does not affect myometrial contraction even in labor.

Pelvic Floor

Pelvic floor is formed by muscles and their fascial coats. The main constituents are pelvic peritoneum, endopelvic fascia, areolar tissue, levator ani muscle, and urogetital diaphragm. The most important of these are endopelvic fascia and levator ani muscle and their fascial coverings.

Levator Ani

Levator ani is a wide sheet of muscle covering the whole of the pelvic floor. Anteriorly it is attached to the back of the pubic bone and posteriorly to the sacrum, coccyx and the anococcygeal raphe on each side. Laterally it is attached to the fascia covering the obturator internus and to the ischial spine. The muscle of each side sweeps downwards and inwards and meet in the midline forming a diaphragm. Three structures, i.e. the urethra anteriorly, vagina in the middle and the rectum posteriorly pass through the muscle. The fascial sheet of the muscle fuses with the fascia covering the vagina and rectum. Levator ani muscle is formed by the following parts .

Pubococcygeus

This is the main part of the muscle. It stretches from the pubis to the coccyx, some part of it also inserts in the perineal body.

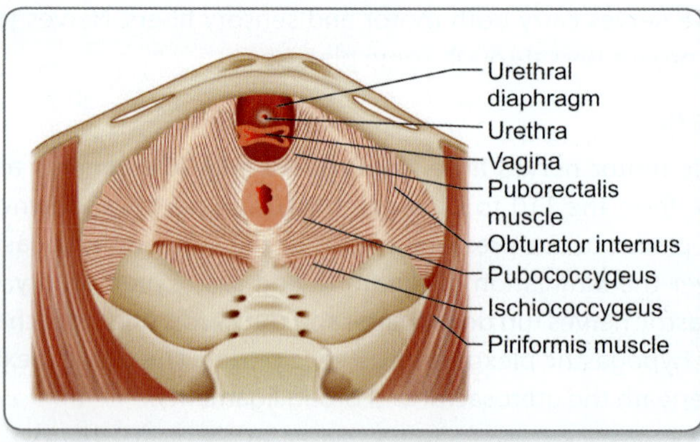

Fig. 11: Pelvic floor, levator ani muscle from above

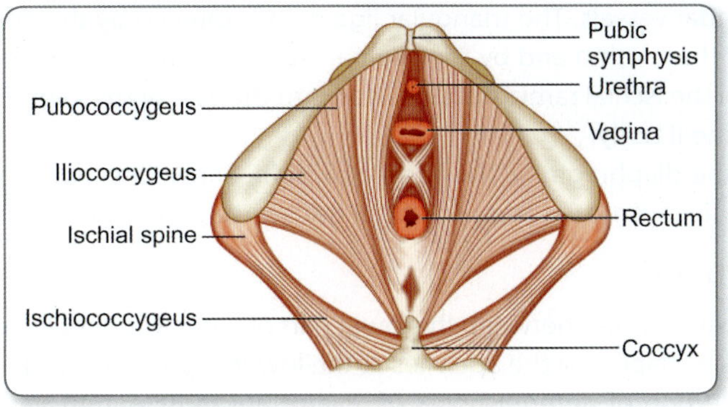

Fig. 12: Levator ani muscle

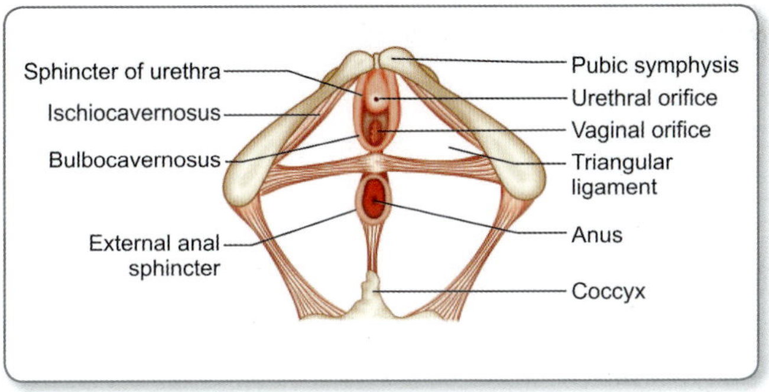

Fig. 13: Superficial perineal muscle

Iliococcygeus

This sheet of muscle stretches from the fascia of obturator internus (white line) to the sacrum, coccyx and anococcygeal raphe. Some part is attached to the perineal body.

Ischiococcygeus

This part arises from the ischial spine and gets inserted in the sacrum and coccyx.

Levator ani is a voluntary muscle. It is supplied by fibers from S3 and S4 roots.

The Triangular Ligament and Perineal Muscles

The triangular ligament or urogenital diaphragm lies below the levator muscle. It is consisted of two layers of fascia, attached anteriorly to the pubic rami. Laterally they are attached to the ischiopubic rami and posteriorly fuse with the central part of perineum. Between the fascial layers lie the compressor urethrae and deep transverse perineal muscles, branches of pudendal nerve and pudendal vessels. The triangular ligament is pierced by the dorsal vein of clitoris, by the urethra and by the vagina. The deep tranverse perineal muscle arises from the ischial rami and is inserted into the wall of the vagina and partly to the perineal body.

Below the diaphragm lie the vestibular bulb, Bartholins gland, bulbospongiosus, ischiocavernosus and superficial transverse perineal muscles.

Perineal Body

The perineal body lies between the lower part of vagina and the anal canal. It is pyramidal in shape and the apex lies at the lower end of rectovaginal septum. Here is insertion of anterior fibers of levator ani muscle, transverse perineal muscle, sphincter vaginae and external sphincter ani muscle. Below the perineal muscles and the perineal body comes the superficial fascia and skin.

chapter 2

Menstruation, Ovulation, Fertilization and Implantation

❐ MENSTRUAL CYCLE

In woman from menarche to menopause is reproductive period. But the best time for reproduction in human is from 21 years of age to 30 years. Thereafter, fertility reduces and after 35 years it reduces substantially. During the reproductive period almost at regular interval there is bleeding from the endometrium, which comes out through the cervix and vagina. This is menstruation. During each menstrual cycle several hormones of the body work in close harmony for the purpose of reproduction.

The Cycle

The menstrual cycle is usually of 28 days. But it may be from 21–35 days.

Period

The bleeding phase continues for 4–6 days. But it may be 2–8 days also which is considered as normal.

Blood Loss

The average blood loss is from 25–60 mL, it may be up to 80 mL.

In women the menstrual cycle is divided into ovarian cycle and uterine cycle. Cycle is again divided into follicular phase and luteal phase. Corresponding with these two phases of ovarian cycles are proliferative phase and secretory phase of the uterine cycle.

Ovarian Cycle

Ovaries produce ovum and secrete female hormones. The process of expulsion of a matured ovum from the surface of the ovary is known as ovulation. Ovulation takes place about 14 days before the next menstruation. But it may vary considerably. During the first-half of the menstrual cycle follicles grow in ovaries and only one grows further to form Graafian follicle which ruptures.

Growth of Follicle and Ovulation

In around 4th week of gestation a part of the coelomic epithelium becomes thick. To this area germ cells migrate from the yolk sac. These germ cells are known as primordial germ cells. The thickened area later develop into gonad.

Primordial germ cells arriving at the gonad differentiate into oogonia. Oogonia continues to undergo cell division by mitosis. Some of them arrest their cell division in prophase of meiosis I and form primary oocyte. Subsequently many oogonia and primary oocyte die becoming atratic. Most of the surviving primary oocyte is surrounded by a layer of flat epithelial cells. The primary oocyte with the surrounding cell layer is called primordial follicle. The arrested process of meiotic division is resumed again at the time of ovulation.

The stromal cells surrounding the granulosa cells also proliferate and arrange in two layers – theca interna and theca externa.

Graafian follicle: Matured primordial follicle is called Graafian follicle. The ovum inside increases in size mainly by increase in amount of cytoplasm. At the same time the amount of liquor follicle increases. The Graafian follicle moves towards the surface of the ovary. Gradually, the follicle projects beyond the surface. At this time the first meiosis is completed, the second meiosis division takes place after ovulation. After these two meiosis divisions the number of chromosome in the ovum become half and two polar bodies are formed. The polar bodies remain in the perivitaline space. Concentration of oestrogen in blood increases with increase in the number of granulosa cells.

The process by which the ovum is extruded from the Graafian follicle is called ovulation. Ovulation is a slow process of escape of the oocyte through a small opening in the follicular wall. The mid cycle LH surge induces increase in prostaglandins and proteolytic enzymes in the follicular walls which make it weak and ultimate perforation of the wall.

Corpus Luteum

After ovulation there is slight bleeding inside the follicle and the walls collapse. There is accumulation of yellow lipid material inside the granulosa cells. The theca cells also become swollen. These are now called theca lutein cells. A corpus luteum is bright yellow in color. A mature corpus luteum is 2–3 cm in diameter. If there is no fertilization of the ovum the corpus luteum starts to

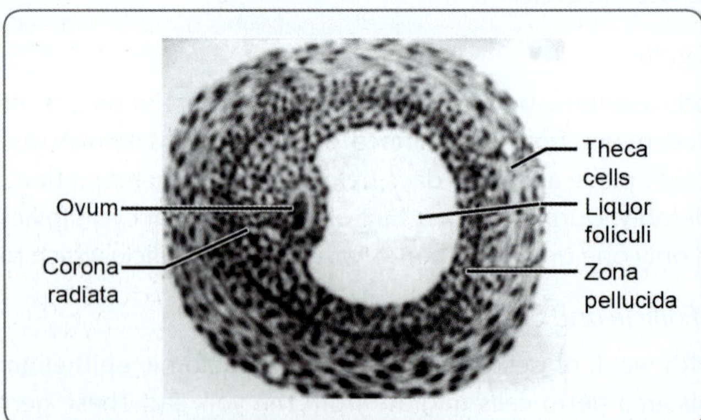

Fig. 1: Graafian follicle

undergo degenerative changes from about 22nd day of menstruation. During the next few weeks it is replaced by white connective tissue and becomes corpus albicans. On the other hand if there is fertilization and pregnancy continues the corpus luteum persists and gradually increases in size.

Endocrinology of menstruation: Gonadotropin releasing hormones (GnRH) are secreted from the hypothalamus. These releasing hormones stimulate the anterior pituitary to secrete follicle stimulating hormone (FSH) and luteinizing hormone (LH). Under the influence of these hormones there is folliculogenesis, ovulation and corpus luteum formation. Under the influence of FSH Graafian follicle is formed from primordial follicle. Oestrogen secreted from growing follicle regulates the secretion of FSH by feedback mechanism. Along with FSH there is secretion of LH in small amount. Just before ovulation there takes place luteinizing hormone surge. Only after luteinizing hormone surge ovulation takes place. After ovulation corpus luteum is formed and secretes both oestrogen and progesterone. Progesterone regulates the secretion of luteinizing hormone. After fertilization the cells of the zygote secrete chorionic gonadotropin hormone which maintains the activity of the corpus luteum.

Endometrial cycle: Growth and development of the endometrium depends on the effects of ovarian hormones—oestrogen and progesteron. The aim of the regular monthly changes in the endometrium is to receive the blastocyst, a change that takes place in fertilized ovum, proper embedding of the blastocyst and continuation of pregnancy. The changes in endometrium are described in two phases – proliferative phase and secretary phase.

Proliferative phase: After menstruation the basal layer of endometrium remains intact. There is re-growth of endometrium from the torn ends of the glands of the basal layer, under the influence of oestrogen. At this stage endometrium is thin and is about 1–2 mm in thickness. From this stage there is gradual growth under the influence of oestrogen. At the early stage the endometrial glands are straight, narrow; stroma is thin and blood vessels are also scanty. Gradually the glands become long and enlarged, the stroma becomes thick and the blood vessels also enlarge in size. In the later part of this

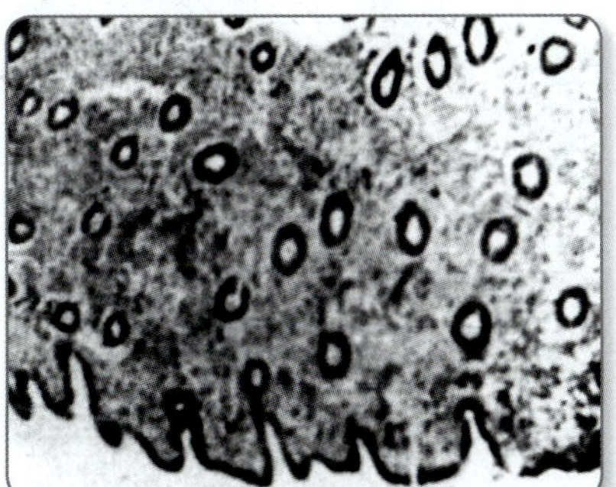

Fig. 2: Endometrium in proliferative phase with tubular glands

phase, i.e. from about 9th – 10th day to 13th day endometrium is about 10 mm in thickness.

Secretary phase: After ovulation corpus luteum secrets oestrogen and progesterone. Progesterone acting on oestrogen primed endometrium brings about secretory change in endometrium. It is called secretory phase because there is secretion of protein-rich fluid inside the glands. The glands enlarge and becomes long. Initially the secretion remains below the nucleus and hence pushes the nucleus to the middle of the gland. At a later stage secretion come out of the cells and push the nucleus to the base again. The length of the glands outgrow the thickness attained by the endometrium, so the glands become tortuous. The stroma become compact and edematus, the blood vessels also enlarge in size and become tortuous, these are called spiral artery. At this stage the endometrium can be divided into three distinct layers—the superficial compact layer, here lies the upper parts of the glands and the thick stroma. The second layer below the first layer is spongy layer. Here lies the enlarged glands, so it looks spongy. The third layer is the basal layer. This layer is not influenced by ovarian hormones and hence remains same. At the later part of this phase sufficient secretion comes out of the glands and blood vessels also grow to a great extent.

Menstrual phase: In the absence of fertilization and implantation the corpus luteum ceases to secrete estrogen and progesterone which is followed by a series of changes leading to menstruation. As a result of withdrawal of sex hormones, there is profound spiral artery spasm leading to endometrial ischaemia. At the same time due to breakdown of lysosomes there is release of proteolytic enzyme which causes destruction of endometrium. This portion of endometrium is shed along with bleeding. Prostaglandin F2α which is a potent vasoconstrictor is released in high concentration during menstruation and causes further vasoconstriction and endometrial destruction. Gradually whole of the endometrium upto the spongy layer is destroyed and is expelled along with blood. This is menstruation. After a portion of the endometrium is shed new epithelium grow from the torn end of the glands and the process

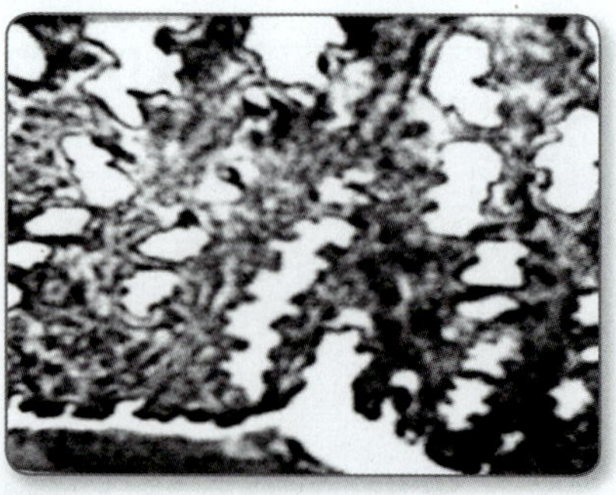

Fig. 3: Endometrium in secretory phase with dilated glands

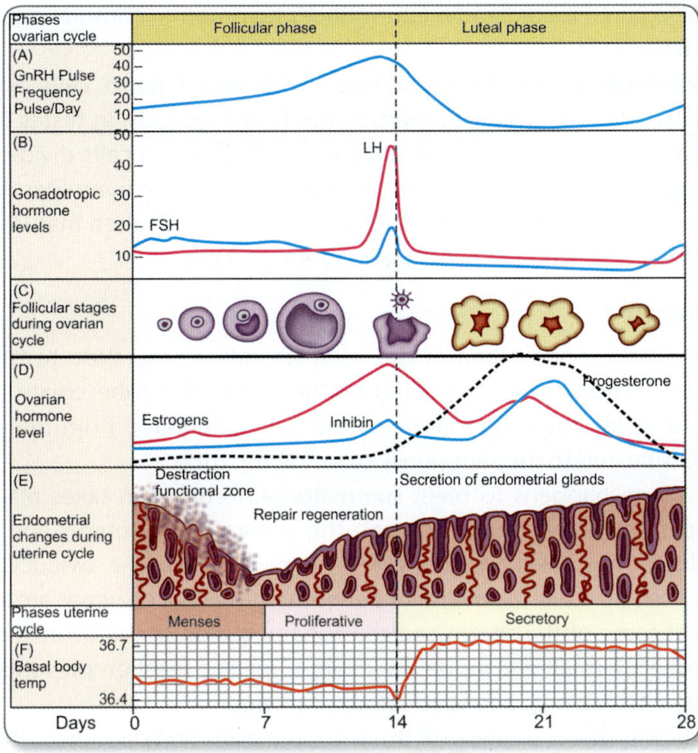

Fig. 4: The menstrual cycle

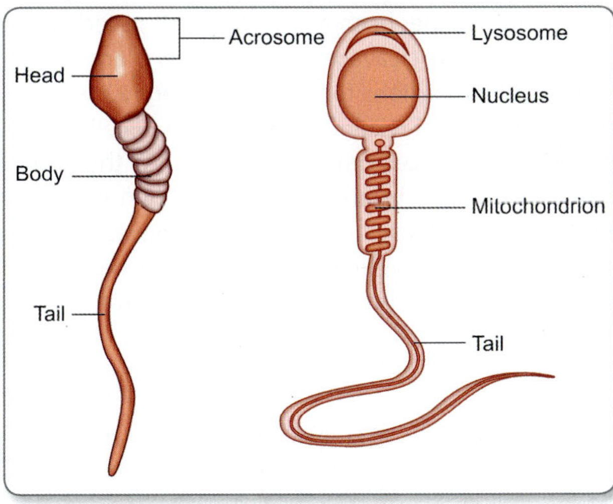

Fig. 5: Spermatozoa

continues again. Prostaglandin F2α induces myometrial contraction also and reduces blood loss.

Spermatozoa are produced in testes. Primordial germ cells appear in the yolk sac and migrate from there to the future gonads. In testes from the primordial germ cells spermatozoa are developed. These cells divide to form spermatogonia and after successive redivisions produce primary spermatocyte, the secondary spermatocyte and spermatids. Spermatids then mature to form spermatozoa. This whole process takes about 72 days.

Fertilization

During ovulation the fimbria of the fallopian tube come close to the ovary. The cilliary movement of the lining epithelium of the tube create a wavey movement inside the tube that helps the ovum, liberated from the ovary to enter the tube and to migrate slowly to inside the tube.

If the ovum happens to meet spermatozoa, fertilization takes place. After coitus, spermatozoa traverses through the cervical canal, uterus and reaches the oviduct. They take minimum 2–7 hours to reach the oviduct. Several spermatozoa surround the ovum for penetration. Several enzymes are liberated by the acrosome of the sperm and the zona pellucida of the ovum. Following entry of one spermatozoa inside the ovum a specific reaction prevents further penetration. Hence only one spermatozoa can enter.

Entry of the sperm triggers off the second maturation division of the ovum. This is followed by fusion of the chromosomes of the ovum and the sperm. Fusion of the chromosomes of ovum and sperm form segmentation nucleus. A segmentation nucleus contains 23 chromosomes from the sperm and 23 from the ovum. So the total number becomes 46. Now it is called zygote.

Following fusion the first cleavage division takes place within 24 hours of fertilization. Subsequent divisions follow about every 22 hours. Cleavage is a series of mitotic division and results in an increase in cells, blastomere. After repeated cell divisions a 16-cell morula is formed. As the morula enters the uterine a small cavity begins to appear inside it. Then it is called blastocyst and the cavity is blastocystic cavity. Cell mass on one side of the cavity forms inner cell mass from which the embryo properly develops. The outer cells which surround the inner cell mass and the cavity form trophoblast. At this

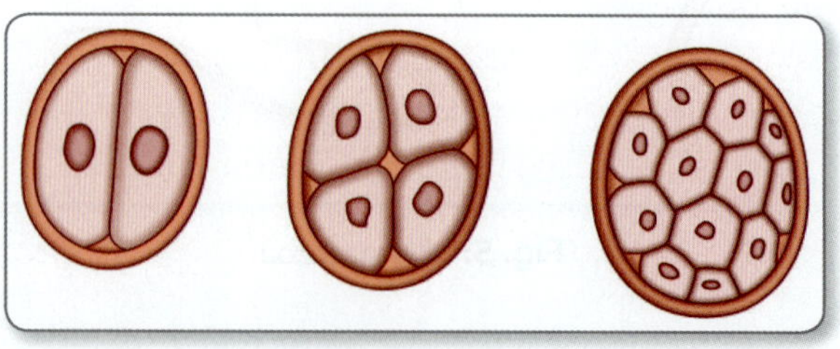

Fig. 6: Cleavage two-cell stage to morula

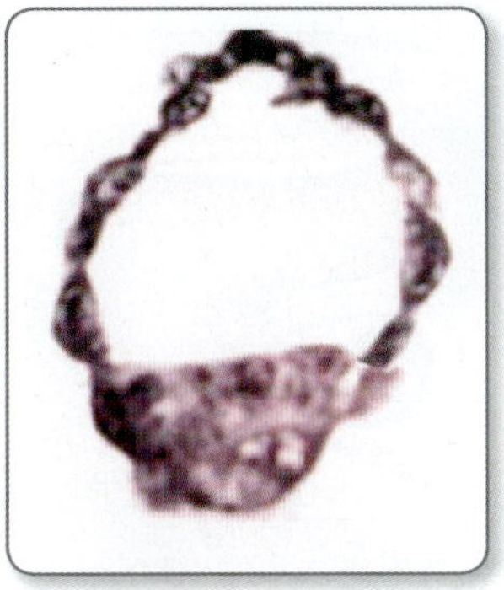

Fig. 7. Blastocyst

stage blastocyst gets embedded into the endometrium, which at this time is in secretary phase.

Implantation

Implantation takes place at blastocyst stage of the embryo. The zona pellucida disappears allowing implantation to begin. The endometrium at the time of implantation is in secretary phase. Normally the human embryo implants on the anterior or posterior wall of the body of the uterus. The blastocyst becomes implanted between the openings of glands.

The trophoblastic cells over the inner cell mass begin to penetrate between the epithelial cells of the endometrium by about sixth post-ovulatory day. Attachment and invasion of the trophoblast are brought by integrins liberated by trophoblast and extracelular matrix molecules laminin and fibronectin. Laminin and fibronectin stimulate attachment and migration respectively. Thus implantation is the result of both trophoblastic and endometrial interaction. Gradually the trophoblast erode deep into the endometrium. The endometrial stroma near the site of implantation is edematous and highly vascular. The large glands secrete abundant glycogen and mucus. By 9th day after fertilization the blastocyst is deeply embedded in the endometrium and the gap on the surface epithelium is sealed by fibrin coagulum. The trophoblast grow and vacuoles appear in the syncytium. When these vacuoles fuse they form large lacunae. After completion of embedding the surface epithelium of endometrium covers the defect in epithelial lining.

At the embryonic pole the lacunar spaces in the syncytio trophoblast form an intercommunicating network. At the same time the trophoblast enters deep into the endometrium and erode the endothelial lining of the dilated vessels—the sinusoids. As the trophoblast erode more and more sinusoids maternal blood begins to flow through these network and uteroplacental circulation begins.

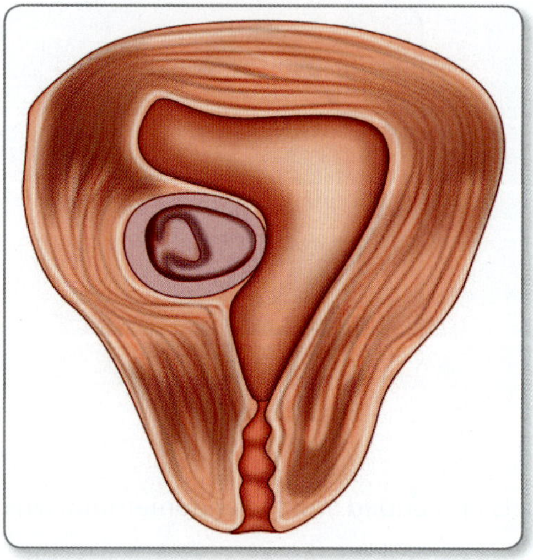

Fig. 8: Developing embryo implented inside the uterine wall

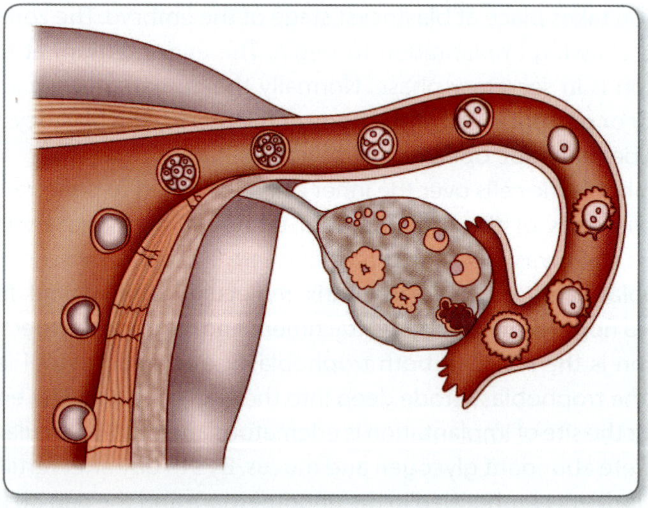

Fig. 9: Ovulation, fertilization, cleavage and implantation

Decidua

Endometrium during pregnancy is called decidua. Blastocyst gets implanted inside this layer. After implantation by hypertrophy of the stromal cells the decidua becomes thicker and more soft. The dilated glands remain in the spongy later. Blastocyst remain in the compact layer, only a small part remain exposed being covered by a layer of surface epithelium of endometrium. In relation to the developing embryo decidua is described in three parts.

Decidua Basalis

The part of decidua between the developing embryo and myometrium is called decidua basalis. Placenta develops in this part.

Decidua Capsularis

The part of decidua covering the embryo inside the uterine cavity is decidua capsularis. Along with increase in size of the embryo decidua capsularis swells up and enlarges in size.

Decidua Vera

Decidua covering the rest of the uterus is called decidua vera. Around twelve weeks of pregnancy when the gestational sac occupies whole of the uterine cavity decidua capsularis blends with decidua vera.

chapter

3 The Fetus

Development of the fetus is described in three phases. The first 2 weeks from conception is termed as zygote or ovular period. From 3–8 weeks it is embryonic period and from 8th week till term is fetal period. For clinical purposes the period of gestation is calculated from the first day of last menstrual period. Embryologist uses the date of ovulation for the same calculation. Students should remember this point while going through this chapter.

During the second month of development the age of the embryo is expressed as crown-rump length (CRL) in millimeters. CRL is measured from the vertex of the skull to the mid-point between the apices of the buttocks. During the 2nd month there is increase in size of the head and formation of the limbs, face, ears, nose and eyes. The ectodermal layer of the trilaminar disc of the embryo gives rise to central nervous system, peripheral nervous system, sensory epithelium of ear, nose and eye, skin, hairs, nail, pituitary gland, mammary and sweat glands, etc. From the mesodermal layer develop muscle tissue, cartilage, bones and subcutaneous tissue. Mesoderm also gives rise to vascular system, urogenital system, spleen, cortex of the suprarenal glands. The endoderm gives rise to epithelial lining of the gastrointestinal tract, respiratory tract, urinary bladder, thyroid and parathyroid glands, liver and pancreas. Organogenesis is completed by the end of 8th week of gestation.

Fetal period is from 9th week to birth: This period of fetal development is marked by maturation of tissues and organs and rapid growth of the body. There is rapid increase in length of the fetus upto 20th week of gestation and weight increases during the last two months.

Fetal development during 8th to 12th week: During this period the face of the fetus becomes more human like. Limbs reach their relative length in comparison with the body. Primary ossification centers appear in long bones and skull; external genitalia develops and loops of intestine withdrawn into the abdominal cavity. By end of 3rd month reflex activities appear.

During 12th to 20th week: The fetus lengthens rapidly and there is little increase in weight. Lanugo hairs appear, head hairs are also visible. During the 5th month movement of the fetus is felt by the mother.

During 21st to 28th week: The skin of the fetus is red in color and wrinkled due to lack of subcutaneous connective tissue. Most of the organs are able to function. Some sounds are heard.

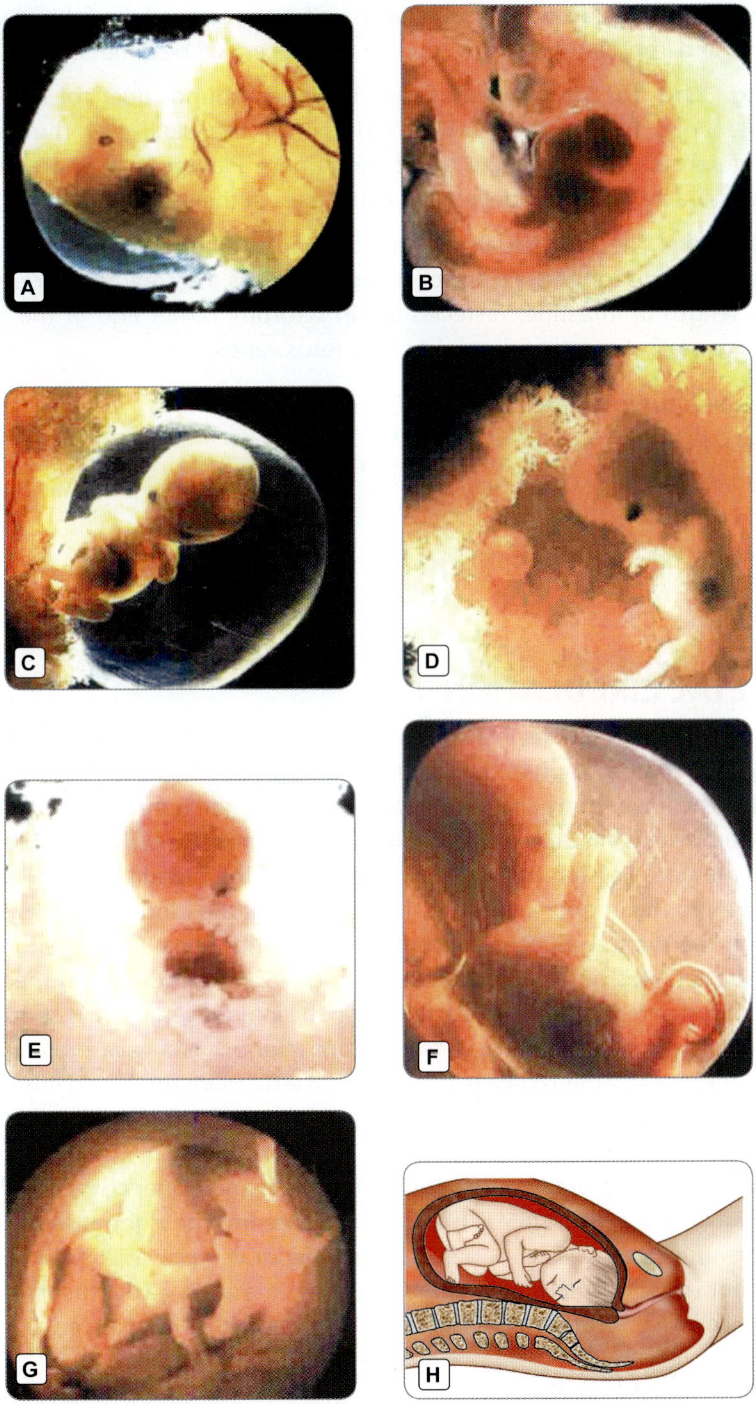

Figs 1A to H: Fetus at different stages of development. (A) Four weeks; (B) Six weeks; (C) Eight weeks; (D) Ten weeks; (E) Twelve weeks; (F) Sixteen weeks; (G) Thirty-two weeks and (H) Term fetus

During 29th to 32nd week: Subcutaneous fat appear and the fetus starts to store fat and iron. Lanugo hairs disappear from face. Skin becomes pale.

During 33rd to 36th week: Fetus becomes round due to increased subcutaneous fat. At the end of 9th month the skull has the largest circumference. Nails reach the tip of the fingers. Planter creases are visible. Sexual characters are well-developed with testes in the scrotum.

At 40 weeks: The nails usually project beyond the fingers. The skin is pink. Lanugo hairs disappears except over the shoulders. Meconium is present in whole length of intestine. Testecles are in scrotum. Lower end of the femur begins to ossify. Length and weight of the fetus varies.

Length of fetus in different period of gestation:

9–12 weeks : 5–8 cm
17–20 weeks : 15–19 cm
25–28 weeks : 24–27 cm
29–32 weeks : 28–30 cm
33–36 weeks : 31–34 cm
37–38 weeks : 35–36 cm

❐ FETAL CIRCULATION

Fetal circulation functions in such a way that maximizes the delivery of more highly oxygenated blood to the upper body and brain, less highly oxygenated blood to the lower body and very low blood flow to the non-functional lungs.

The umbilical vein carrying oxygenated blood (about 80%) from the placenta enters the portal system of the fetus. A portion of the blood pass through the liver, then to the inferior vena cava. The majority of the blood bypass the liver through the ductus venosus and enters the inferior vena cava. Inferior vena cava also receives unsaturated venous blood (25% saturated) from the lower limbs. Blood entering into the heart through the inferior vena cava is about 70% oxygenated. About one-third of blood from inferior vena cava preferentially pass across the foramen ovale to left atrium. In left atrium this blood mixes with the small amount of blood from the pulmonary vein. From left atrium blood flows to the left ventricle and then to the ascending aorta.

Branches from proximal aorta supply the brain and upper part of the body with highly oxygenated (65%) blood. Blood entering the right atrium via the inferior vena cava mixes with blood from superior vena cava (25% saturated). Blood from right ventricle (55% saturated) enters the aorta via ductus arteriosus. The descending aorta supplies the lower body (about 60% saturated).

Changes After Birth

Something important happens within the baby after birth. Baby takes respiration immediately after birth, which inflates the lungs. Following inflation blood

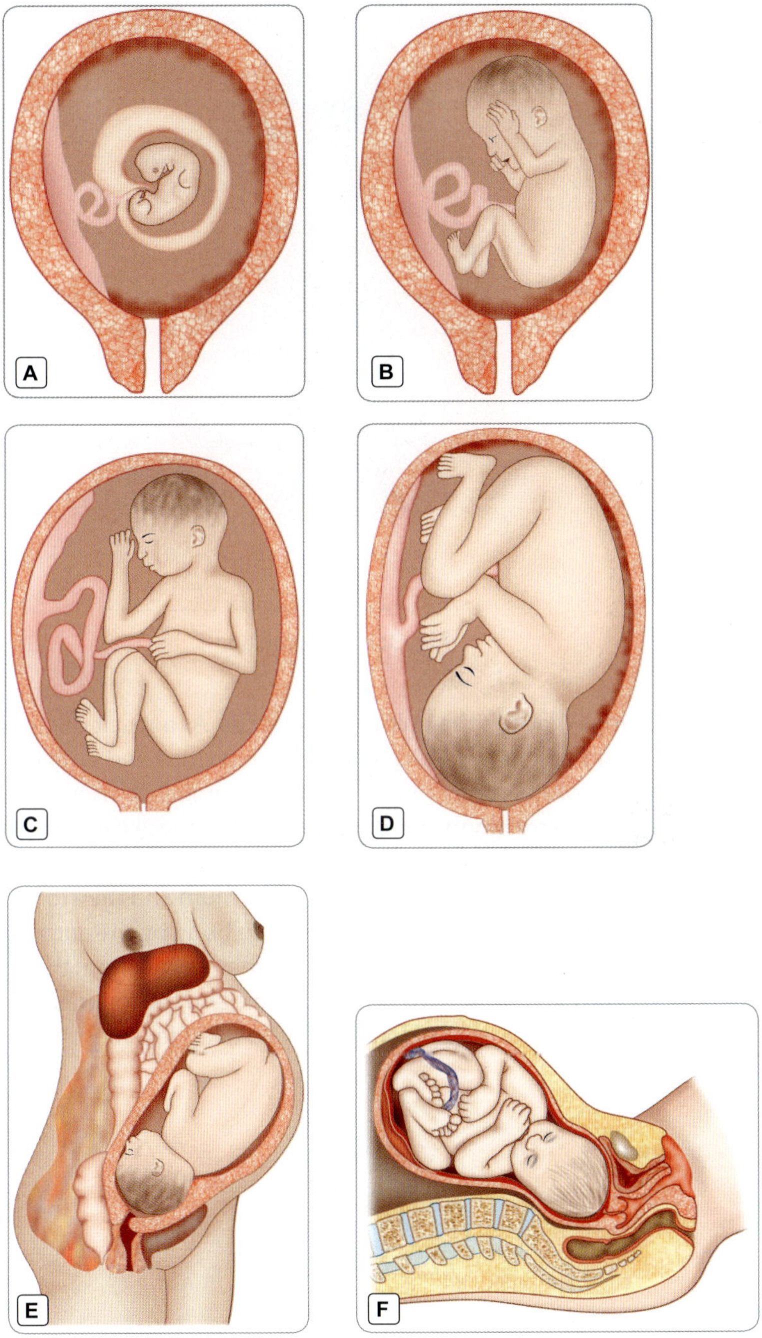

Figs 2A to F: Fetus inside uterus in different periods of gestation. (A) Six weeks; (B) Eight weeks; (C) Twelve weeks; (D) Twenty eight weeks; (E) Thirty-six weeks and (F) Full term fetus

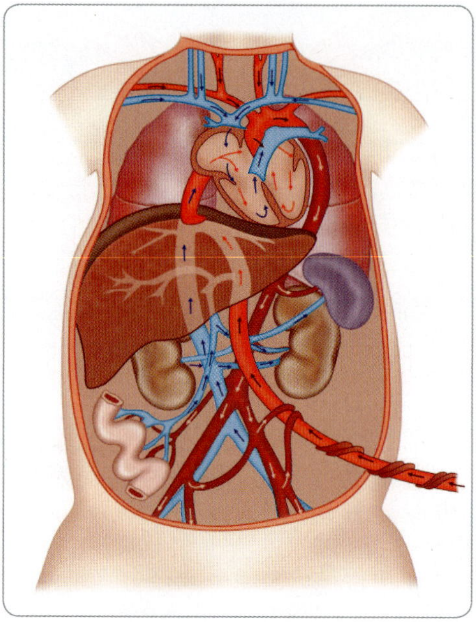

Fig. 3: Fetal circulation

rush to the lungs through the pulmonary arteries. As a result ductus arteriosus closes down and obliterates. Placental circulation stops and umbilical vein and ductus venosus collapse and then obliterate. The umbilical arteries (hypogastric arteries) no more carry blood and collapse. In adult these can be recognized as obliterated hypogastric arteries.

Oxygenated blood return from lungs to left atrium and then to left ventricle. This oxygenated blood is supplied to the whole body by the aorta. Blood from atriums enters the ventricles of both sides. No more blood from the right atrium enters the left atrium through the foramen ovale and the foramen closes down. Complete anatomical closure of foramen ovale takes few months.

chapter

4 Development of Placenta

Fertilization is the process of union of male and female gametes. Fertilization is followed by a series of cell divisions forming a mass of cells known as morula. Then there is fluid collection forming a single fluid filled cavity known as blastocyst. At one side of the cyst there is concentration of cells called inner cell mass, the other side is lined by a single layer of flat cells. By this time zona pellucida covering the ovum disappear. The fertilized ovum takes about 3 days to reach the endometrical cavity.

Inside the uterine cavity the embryo undergoes further development. After zona is shed the blastocyst adhers to the endometrium. Some proteolytic enzymes help in this process. When the blastocyst contacts the endometrium for implantation, syncytiotrophoblast appear. It is a sheet of cellular material studded with nuclei without cell wall. The syncytiotrophoblast is thought to be formed by breaking down of the cell wall of the cytotrophoblast. Subsequent mitotic activity and DNA synthesis occur in the nuclei of cytotrophoblast only. Syncytiotrophoblast differentiate from cytotrophoblast. At about 9th day fluid-like spaces appear within the syncytiotrophoblast. This is soon followed by appearance of the maternal blood due to erosion of endometrial capillaries and fill the lacunae. These lacunae soon become confluent and form the future intervillous space. Syncytial trophoblast grow in trabecular column. They grow all around with a central cytotrophoblastic core. Cytotrophoblast continue to grow into the decidua and become attached there. By this time a mesenchymal core appear within the villous stem. Later vessels develop there in situ.

The villous stem formed by the cytotrophoblastic cells goes deeper and anchore to the decidua of the basal plate. Sprouts appear from the primary

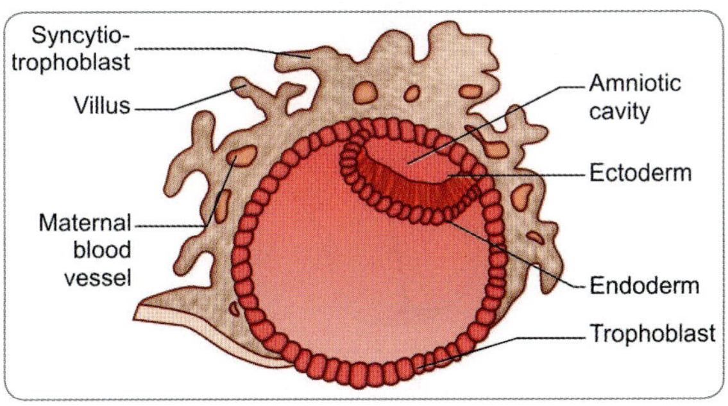

Fig. 1: Germinal layers with formation of villi

villous stem. At the initial stage they are consisted of syncytiotrophoblast only, gradually they pass through the stages of intrusion of cytotropoblast, formation of mesenchyme and then vascularization. These are primary stem villi. These are true villi. By 21st post-ovulatory day the placenta is a vascularized villous organ. The primary stem villi grow and give rise to secondary and tertiary stem villi. Later on these break up into the terminal villous tree. From this time till the end of 60th week of pregnancy placenta continues to grow.

The villi over the gestational sac towards the uterine cavity degenerate and form chorion leave, and the thin rim of decidua covering it gradually disappear. The chorion leave come in contact with the decidua of the opposite uterine wall. The villi towards the decidual plate proliferate and form the chorion frondosum and develop into a definitive placenta.

During the 3rd month of gestation placental septa grow into the intervillous space from the basal plate. They divide the maternal surface of the placenta into 15–20 lobes. Septas are formed by remnants of trophoblastic cells imbedded in fibrinoid material. These septa have no physiological role. By the end of 4th month of gestation placenta achieves its definitive form but growth continues

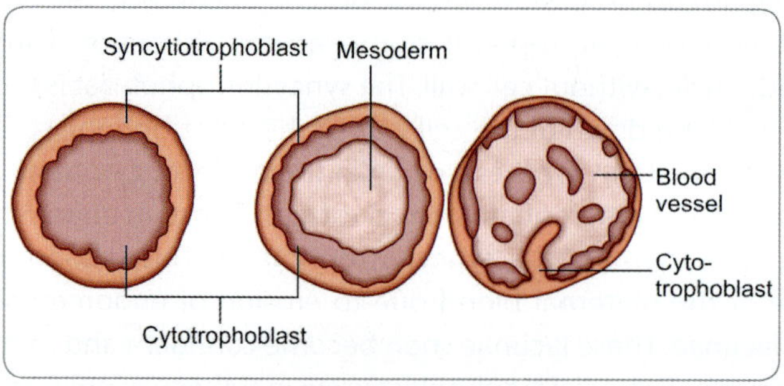

Fig. 2: Showing different stages of villus formation

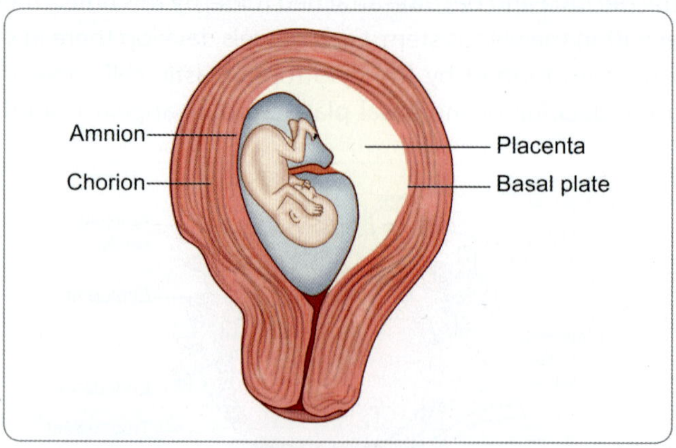

Fig. 3: Relation of placenta with fetal membranes

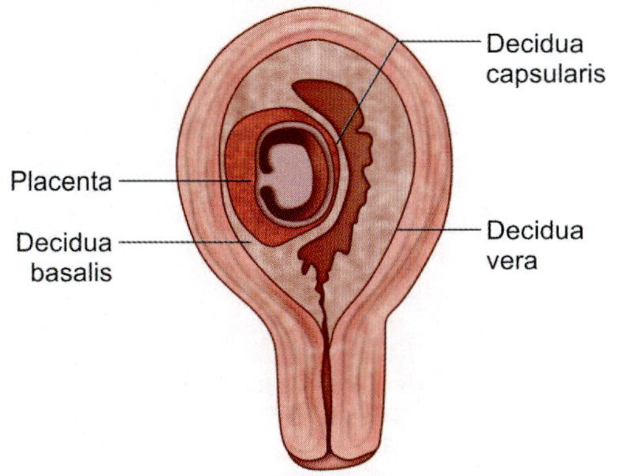

Fig. 4: Relation of placenta with decidua

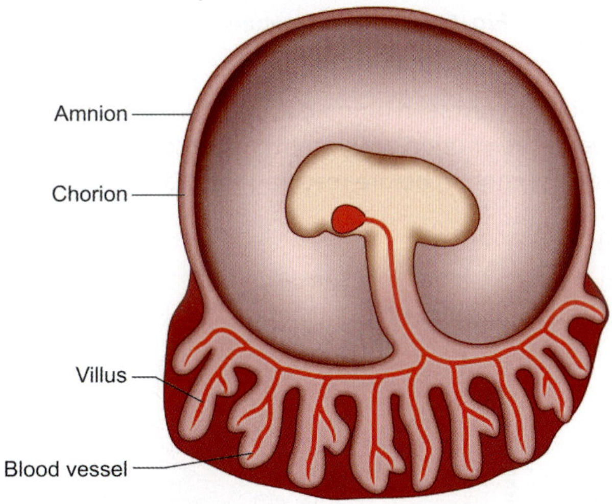

Fig. 5: Formation of placenta and fetal membranes

till term. This growth is due to formation of new villi and branching of the villous tree.

❐ FETAL MEMBRANES

Fetal membranes are two in number, chorion outside and amnion inside.

The Chorion

After formation of placenta the rest of the chorion atrophies and remains as a thin membrane between decidua outside and amnion inside. Sometimes

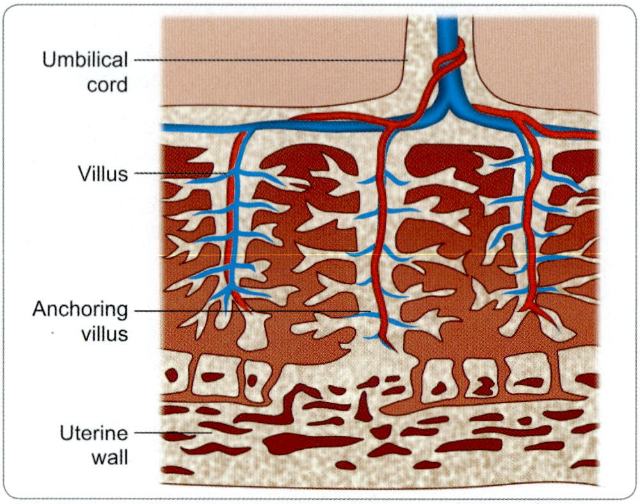

Fig. 6: Structure of matured placenta

vessels from umbilical cord seen running across it. In velamentous insertion the cord is attached to the chorion away from the placenta and umbilical arteries and veins run across chorian before reaching the placenta.

Abnormality of Placenta

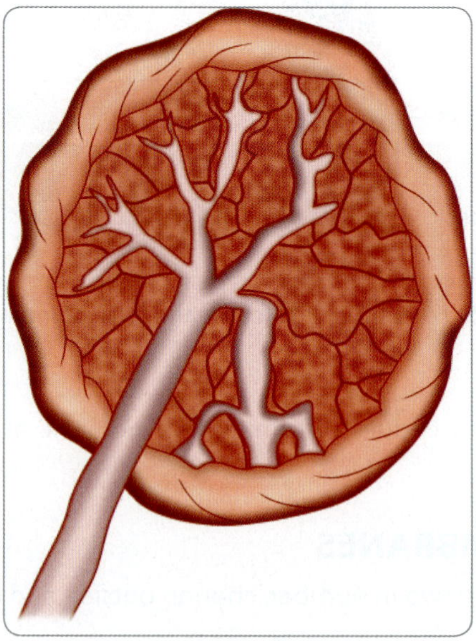

Fig. 7: Circumvalet placenta

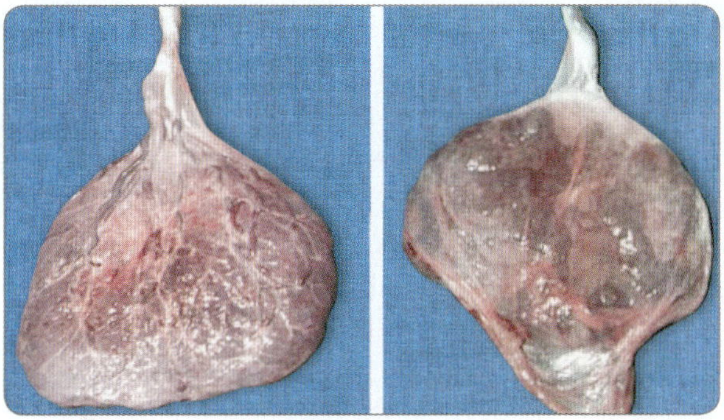

Fig. 8: Battledore placenta

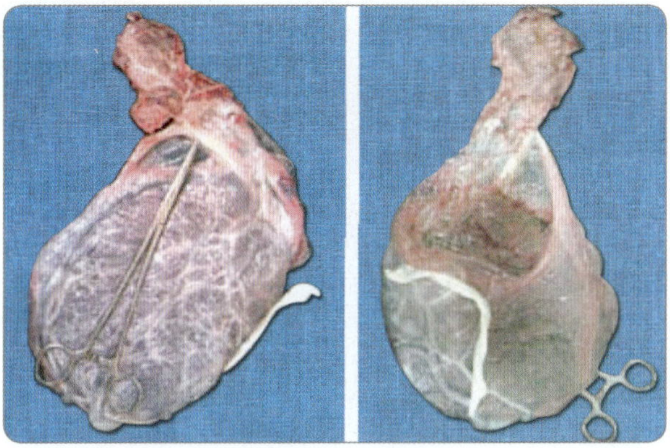

Fig. 9: Succenturiate placenta

The Amnion

The inner cell mass by 8th and 9th post-ovulatory day form the bilaminar disc. The layer of cells facing the blastocystic cavity is embryonic endoderm and the outer layer is embryonic ectoderm. Amniotic cavity appears between the embryonic ectoderm and trophoblast. Endodermal cells line the blastocystic cavity and form yolk sac. Extra embryonic coelom appears in the extra embryonic mesenchyme. It enlarges and separates the amnion from the inner aspect of the chorion. Subsequently the amniotic cavity enlarges. The developing embryo projects into the amniotic cavity. Gradually there is further expansion of the amniotic cavity obliterating the extra embryonic coelom. The embryo is carried into the amniotic cavity by elongation of the umbilical cord which is completely covered by the amnion. The amnion is also loosely attached to the placenta and chorion. They can be separated easily from one another upto the insertion of the umbilical cord.

Histologically amniochorion consists of a single layer of flat or cubical epithelium. These cells contain granules, fat droplets and vacuoles. The next layer, the connective tissue is closely applied to similar connective tissue of chorion. Few trophoblastic cells may be present in chorion.

❒ UMBILICAL CORD

The umbilical cord forms the connection between the fetus and the placenta. It is derived from the body stalk. It consists of two arteries and a vein embedded in Wharton's jelly. It is covered by a single layer of epithelium of amnion. Wharton's jelly is composed of abundant gelatinous material, rich in mucopolysaccharides, collagen fibers, mast cell and few stellate cells. It has a cushioning effect to protect the umbilical vessels from trauma.

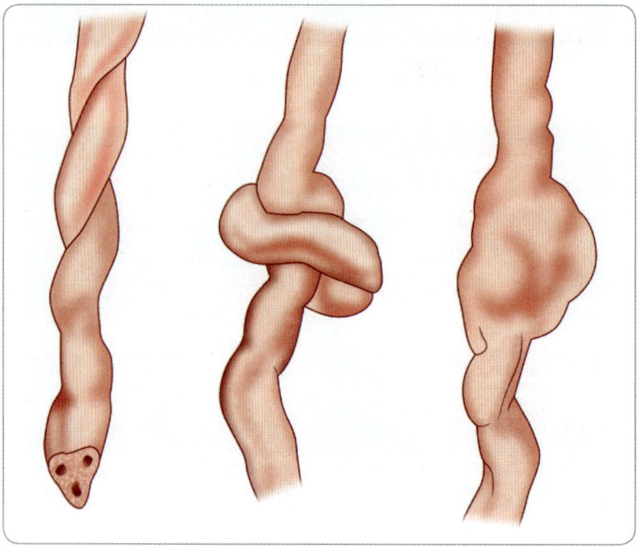

Fig. 10: Umbilical cord (from left) normal, true knot, false knot

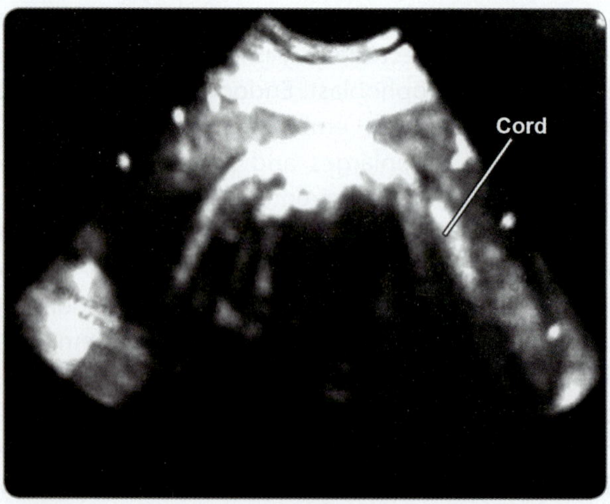

Fig. 11: Ultrasonography showing cord round the neck

The cord is about 50–60 cm long, but the length varies greatly. Male babies tend to have longer cords than the female babies. Thickness of the cord is not uniform as very often it presents with nodes, swelling which are caused by either dilatation of vein or local increase in Wharton's jelly. A long cord predisposes to cord prolapse or torsion and knotting of the cord. Rarely the cord contains one or more true knot due to the fetus passing through a loop of the cord. If the knot becomes tight blood circulation to the fetus is obstructed and the fetus may die in utero. The cord facilitates movement of water and other substances between the fetus and the amniotic fluid. The site of insertion of the cord is usually central, but it may vary widely without any clinical significance.

❐ AMNIOTIC FLUID

Amniotic fluid occupies the amniotic cavity where the growing fetus can move easily. Origin of liquor amnii is still not clear. It is a mixture of both maternal and fetal origin. It is thought to be a transudate from maternal plasma across the fetal membrane particularly covering the placenta and the umbilical cord or a secretion from the amniotic epithelium. Fetal contribution is in the form of fetal urine which is of small amount. Amniotic fluid is usually slightly turbid. Turbidity might be due to presence of solid particles desquamated from fetal skin and amniotic epithelium.

In the early part of pregnancy amniotic fluid is almost like transudate from maternal plasma but during the later part of pregnancy composition changes. At term its specific gravity is about 1010. The inorganic salts it contains are mostly alkaline chlorides, phosphates, sulphates and albumin. Urea, uric acid and creatinine are also present. The solid matters are composed of lanugo hair, epithelial cells, sebaceous materials from fetal skin and cast off amniotic epithelial cells.

The amount of liquor amnii varies greatly according to period of gestation. At term pregnancy the average amount is about 600 mL, the range being from 300–1500 mL. Liquor amnii is in a dynamic state. It is being always exchanged with maternal plasma. At term the whole amount is exchanged in 2.9 hours.

Functions of Liquor Amnii

Liquor amnii provides a protective medium for the fetus against external injury. It equalizes the intrauterine pressure during uterine contraction and provides enough room particularly in mid-pregnancy, for free movement of the fetus. The fetus swallows some liquor which supply some water to the fetus. During labor the bag of forewater helps in dilatation of the cervix. When the membranes rupture during labor it flushes the birth canal from above downwards with a fluid which is aseptic, thereby preventing ascending infection.

Being a fetal component the volume of liquor amnii, its color and concentration of different constituents reflect fetal condition in utero. In today's obstetric practice study of amniotic fluid plays an important role in antenatal assessment of fetal well-being.

chapter

5 Types of Pelvis

There are four types of pelvis described as follows:

❒ GYNECOID

It has a rounded or slightly ovoid inlet, round forepelvis, posterior segment of the pelvis is adequate, sacrum is hollow and inclined backward, straight sidewalls with wide interspinous diameter. Subpubic arch is wide.

❒ ANDROID

In this type inlet is wedge-shaped with narrow forepelvis and flat posterior segment. Sacrum is inclined forward. The side walls converse and subpubic angle is narrow.

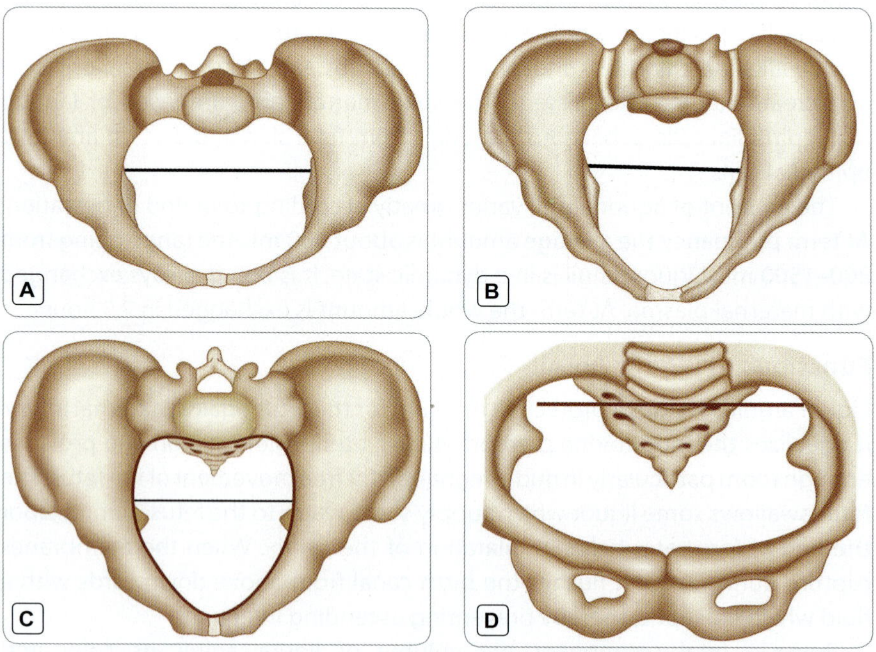

Figs 1A to D: Different types of female pelvis. (A) Gynecoid; (B) Android; (C) Anthropoid and (D) Platypeloid pelvis

❒ ANTHROPOID

The anthropoid pelvis is characterized by a long narrow oval inlet. Anterior and posterior segments are extended and narrow. Sacrum is long and narrow. Side walls are straight but interspinous diameter is narrow.

❒ PLATYPELLOID

In platypelloid pelvis inlet is very wide and oval. Anterior and posterior segments are wide. Sacrum is often flat with normal inclination. Subpubic arch is very wide.

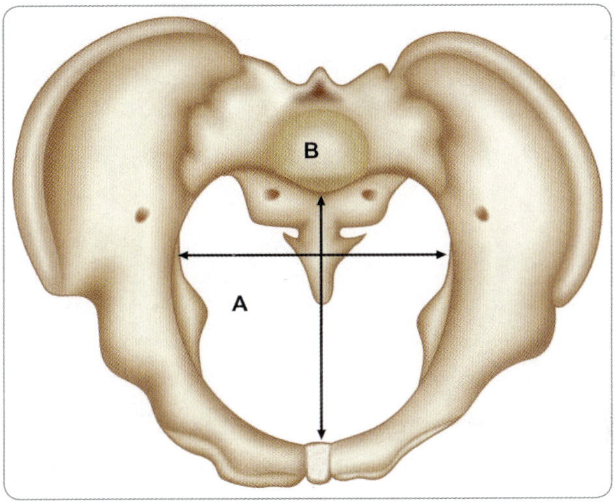

Fig. 2: Diameters of pelvic inlet. (A) anteroposterior and (B) transverse

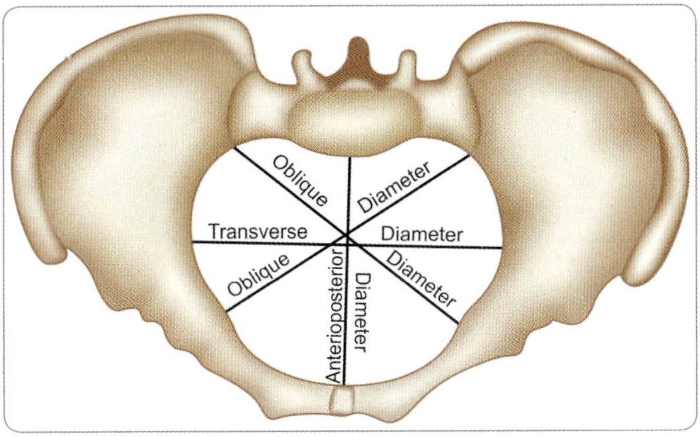

Fig. 3: Different diameters of pelvic inlet

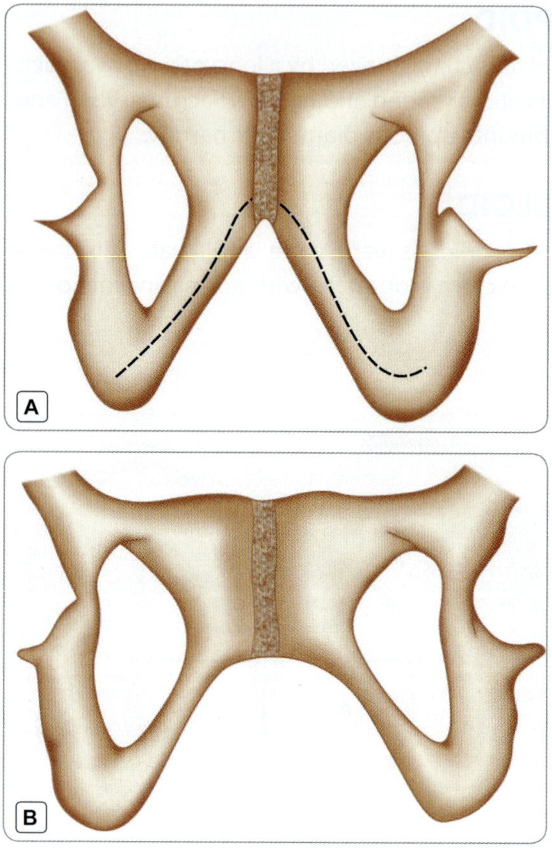

Figs 4A and B: Sub-pubic angle: (A) narrow; (B) wide

chapter

6 Congenital Malformation of Female Genital Tract

Error in development of the female genital tract may give rise to certain interesting conditions. A young girl usually accompanied by her mother comes to gynecologist with some specific complaints related to malformation of genital tract. These malformations can be described in following categories:

❒ CONGENITAL ANOMALIES OF VULVA

Different varities of congenital anomaly may be seen. Ambiguous genitalia very often creates problem to assign sex of the newborn without further evaluation. There may be clitoromegaly, bifid clitoris or midline fusion of labioscrotal fold. Very rarely incomplete development of genitalia may result in a cloaca without separation of urinary bladder and vagina.

Masculinization of a female fetus in utero leads to female pseudohermophroditism. Masculinization of the genetically female fetus may result from congenital adrenal hyperplasia or from exogenous hormone ingestion by the mother. On examination clitoris is found to be enlarged, there may be various degree of fusion of labioscrotal folds producing hypospadias. Internal genital organs are usually normal.

On the other hand a genetically male fetus may present with complete external phenotypic development of female. This occurs in testicular feminization. Male pseudohermophroditism is commonly the result of genetic mosaicism. In this condition there may be varying degree of virilization and Müllerian development.

In dealing with such a situation few things are important to come to a diagnosis. These include careful physical examination, pelvic ultrasonography, buccal smear for sex chromatin, hormone assay and karyotyping. Sometimes gonadal biopsy may be needed to evaluate the nature of the gonad.

❒ VAGINA

Few developmental anomalies of vagina may be encountered.

Imperforated Hymen

This is the mildest form of canalization abnormality. It blocks the lower most part of the vagina where the vaginal plate contacts the urogenital sinus.

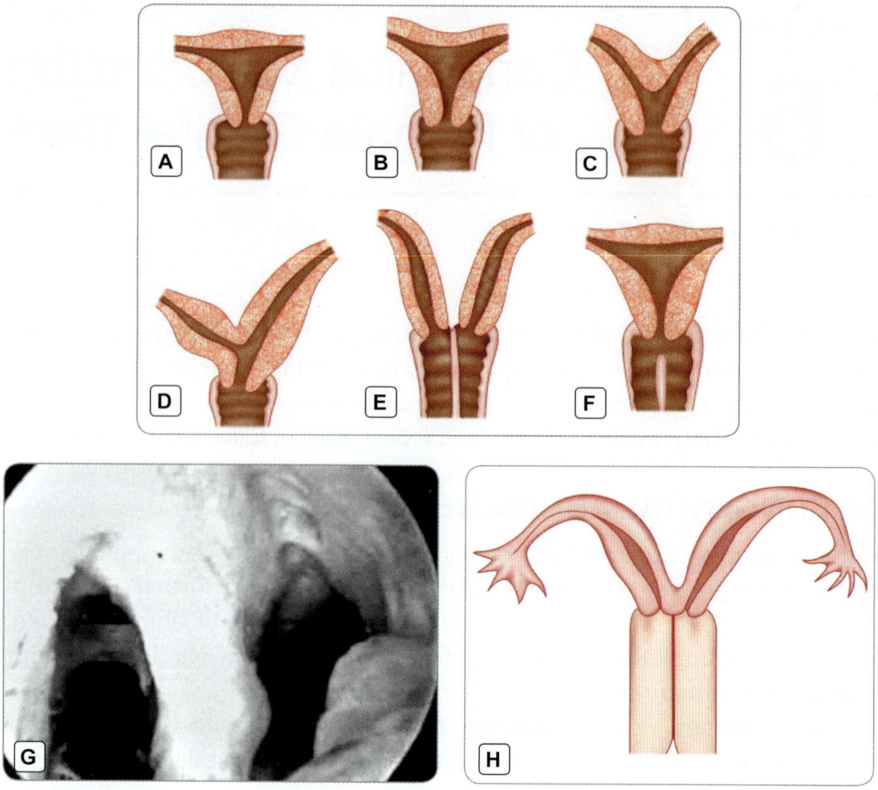

Figs 1A to H: Uterine abnormalities. (A), (B) Arcuate uterus; (C) Bicornuate; (D) Bicornuate uterus with rudimentary horn; (E) Uterus didelphys; (F) Septate vagina; (G) Uterine septa (hysteroscopic view); (H) Double uterus, double cervix and double vagina

Midline Longitudinal Septum

Midline longitudinal septum creats double vagina. This septa is usually associated with double cervix and double uterus called uterus didelphys.

Vaginal agenesis or absence of vagina is a rare condition. If the uterus is also absent with normal fallopian tubes and ovaries the defect is Müllerian agenesis or Mayer-Rokitansky-Küster-Hauser syndrome.

Gartner's duct cyst

It arises from the remnant of the Walffian duct, the size varying from 1–5 cm. In the upper part of vagina, they are found on the anterolateral wall and more laterally in the lower vagina. They usually remain asymptomatic.

Developmental Anomaly of Uterus and Cervix

The upper vagina, cervix, uterus and fallopian tubes develop from the paramesonephric duct (Muiillerian duct). By the 6th week of gestation genital ridge develops as a prominent swelling on the medial side of the mesonephros. This is future ovary. Germ cells appear in the yolk sac and migrate actively from the hind gut, through the mesentary and the dorsal body wall, into the genital ridge. At the same time the paramesonephric ducts or Müllerian ducts appear lateral to the mesonephric ducts. They grow caudally and then medially to fuse in the midline. In pelvis they contact the urogenital sinus behind the region of the urethra and form a thickening—sinusal tubercle. Finally this solid rod of cells canalizes. This passage is the utero vaginal canal. The sinusal tubercle indicates the position of the hymen. The part of the urogenital sinus above it forms the urethra and the part below widens to form the vestibule where both urethra and vagina open.

Developmental Anomaly of the Uterus

The common uterine anomalies are due to failure of the process of canalization of the Müllerian cords or due to incomplete fusion of the Müllerian ducts or due to formation failure.

❒ FAILURE OF CANALIZATION OF THE MÜLLERIAN CORDS

Incomplete canalization of the Müllerian cord results in absence of vagina. Usually the part of vagina just below the cervix remains unaffected. In many cases the lower part of the vagina may remain noncanalized.

Defect in Fusion of the Müllerian Duct

Different types of anomaly may develop from defective fusion of two halves of Müllerian ducts.

Uterus Didelphys

In this condition there is complete absence of fusion of two Müllerian ducts. There are two uterus, two cervix and two vagina. Each half of the uterus has its own fallopian tube and ovary.

Uterus Bicornis Bicollis

In this condition, the two halves of uterus remain completely separated and cervix is also divided into two by a septum (Fig. 1E).

Uterus Bicornis unicollis

In this condition, the body of the uterus is divided but cervix is normal. Both the horns of uterus communicate with the cervix.

Uterus Unicornis

In uterus unicornis only one-half of the Müllerian duct develops to produce one uterus, one fallopian tube and one vagina. The other-half may remain in a rudimentary form with or without a patent canal. This horn usually is not communicated with cervix. A patent, functional cavity leads to hematometra after menstruation begins.

Septate Uterus

In this condition fusion is complete but internally the cavity of the uterus is partly or completely subdivided into two halves by a midline septum. Sometimes vagina may also have a septum.

In some women, the cervix may be congenitally elongated. Elongation is confined to the vaginal portion of the cervix.

chapter

7 History Taking

As in other branches of Medicine in Obstetrics and Gynecology also history taking is the first step towards diagnosis. To arrive at a correct diagnosis history taking is followed by physical examination and necessary laboratory investigations.

History taking is nothing short of an art. The techniques of history taking should be cultivated by every student of Medicine. In obstetrics the doctor deals with a group of women during their most sensitive period of life. Similarly gynecology is a subject dealing with diseases of female generative organs. As such it involves some personal and most private issues of the couple. Therefore, the approach of the doctor should be reassuring and comforting to the women.

Minute observation and patient hearing to the problems are important. Students of medical science should try to train their sensory organs, e.g. to see, to touch, to smell, to listen and to perceive the problems of the woman. History taking as a whole is a comprehensive method to know the woman and her family. A favorable doctor-patient relationship is essential to achieve full confidence of the woman and to have a free communication with her. An open and free communication is needed to elicit the complete history. A complete history includes the woman, her family, the environment, her dietary habit, sexual life and her social background. In other words the woman should be considered as a whole. The art of developing proper communication with the woman needs practice. The patient should be allowed to tell her story in her own words, though many a times it may be vague and evasive one. The doctor should listen to her patiently. This would make the patient at her ease and then it becomes easy for the doctor to gain her confidence. Another important point the doctor should keep in mind is the type of woman he is dealing with. She might be illiterate or of very low intelligence. Sometimes it may be difficult for her to express herself fully.

To elicit a complete history she needs help and encouragement from the doctor. One easy way to gain the confidence of the woman (particularly a woman from a rural area of lower educational strata) is to converse with her in her own language. It is more effective for a free communication. When the woman finishes her story, leading questions should be asked gradually. But care should be taken that the questions in no way embarrass the woman. Because it is well known that in our society the subject relating to sex and child bearing is shrouded by taboos and the woman might be very reluctant to speak every thing. This reluctance might be more pronounced when the doctor is male. A pleasant and sympathetic approach of the doctor to the patients problem is helpful in overcoming this difficulty.

The doctor should freely answer all the questions of the patient and her relatives. It is expected of him to explain the discomfort of the patient, the need of specific laboratory examination and the expected line of management. A smiling face and sympathetic words of a doctor is very much reassuring for the patients. Above all a positive approach of the doctor towards a patient's sufferings is essential and a young doctor should cultivate this habit from the beginning.

It is necessary to realize that history/case note is not finished at the first sitting, rather, it is the beginning. During subsequent visits or in hospital ward note should be taken of new complaints and progress or otherwise of the condition of the patient.

❐ HISTORY IS TAKEN UNDER THE FOLLOWING HEADINGS

1. Identification of the woman.
2. Complaints.
3. Menstrual history.
4. Past history of medical and/or surgical disorder with history of any operation including gynecological operation.
5. Personal history and psychological history, if any.
6. Family history.
7. Past obstetric history.
8. History of drug used during the pregnancy in question.
9. History of use of contraceptives.

Before discussing the details of history taking a few things are worth mentioning. The points made above might not hold true for all patients. For instance, in a primigravida case there will be no past obstetric history, whereas in multiparous women with pregnancy wastage a detailed past obstetric history should be elicited. Again in a primigravida case and in cases with history of infertility duration of marriage should be asked though it may not be so important in a nulliparous woman. Only with experience and practice the doctor will learn to select the points to be concentrated on, in a particular case.

Name

Full name of the patient should be written in block letters followed by the name of the husband or the guardian with full address. It is necessary to know the locality from which the patient has come, for future communication, if needed.

Age

Exact age of the patient should be noted. Though reproductive period spans from menarche to menopause, the most fertile period in a woman's life is from 20–30 years of age beyond which fertility decreases and there is a sharp fall after 35 years of age. Complications during pregnancy and child birth are more common in a woman after 35 years of age. When a woman becomes pregnant for the first time after 35 years of age, she is known as elderly primigravida. Similarly young pregnant woman, i.e. before 18 years of age, present themselves with complication like pregnancy induced hypertension, intrauterine growth restriction, etc. During labor also incidence of operative interference is more in both young and elderly primigravida. In gynecology certain diseases are more common in certain age group. Menstrual abnormalities and sexually transmitted diseases are common during reproductive age group, whereas genital malignancies are common in elderly woman.

Marital Status

Marital status of the woman should be noted as unmarried, married or widow. Pregnancy in unmarried woman or widow may create some problems. These women are usually neglected and they themselves neglect the pregnancy and suffer from nutritional deprivation leading to other complications. Moreover, an unwanted pregnancy may be a source of psychological stress, which may lead to psychosis during pregnancy, or after delivery.

Religion

Religion as such has very little influence on the course of pregnancy and labor. In some rare situations where women constantly remain under cover-purdha and these women may suffer from osteomalacia due to lack of vitamin D. Osteomalacia leads to bony deformity of the pelvis. This condition is rare nowadays. Incidence of high multiparity is more in those communities where sterilization operation is prohibited.

Similarly it has no definite influence in gynecology though it is thought that carcinoma of cervix is less common among Mohammedan due to compulsory circumcision of male. Polygamy and early marriage are thought to be influencing factor for carcinoma of cervix.

Occupation

Occupation of the woman should be mentioned as housewife, industrial worker, office goers, teacher, etc. Most of our woman population are housewives, but with increasing urbanization and growth in industrial activities the number of woman engaged as industrial, office goers and teachers are increasing. Contact with the outside world and their work in factories and offices have some impact on the course of pregnancy, labor and subsequent rearing of the newborn.

In chronic gynecological condition that makes the women incapacitated to attend her regular job is bound to reduce her working hours. This should be noted in case note.

Presenting Complaint(s)

Complaint of the patient should be written in chronological order. Very often a woman does not give history of amenorrhea voluntarily, only on being asked leading questions she does reveal her menstrual history. In early weeks of pregnancy most of the patients come to doctor for diagnosis of pregnancy with history of amenorrhea only. In later part of pregnancy they come for check-up or only when some complaints are there. The complaints should be carefully noted. Besides history of amenorrhea pain abdomen is a common complaint during pregnancy. The points of importance of different complaints are as follows:

Pain

- How long the pain is there
- The exact site of origin of pain
- Whether there is radiation to any other site
- Character of pain – dull aching, spasmodic, pinching
- Continuous or intermittent or occasional
- Whether pain is associated with hardening of the uterus
- Any relation with micturition
- Any relation with posture
- Any relation with food and fetal movement.

Frequency of Micturition

- Duration
- Whether associated with pain or burning sensation
- How often she has to pass urine and what is the amount.

White Discharge

- Duration
- Whether associated with itching of vulva or burning
- Character of the discharge—thick or watery
- Foul smelling or not
- Whether stain her under clothing.

Nausea and Vomiting

- History of hyperacidity
- Frequency, if there is vomiting
- Relation with food
- Contents of vomitus.

Vaginal Bleeding

- Onset—whether sudden, heavy bleeding
- Duration of pregnancy when bleeding occurs
- Amount of bleeding—just spotting or necessitated vaginal pad
- If sanitary pad is used the number of pad needed per day
- Whether associated with pain abdomen
- Any movement that may initiate or aggravate bleeding.

Other Vaginal Discharge

- Vaginal bleeding may be followed by sanguineous discharge or without vaginal bleeding also, there may be brownish watery discharge.
- Presence of sanguineous discharge is characteristic of hydatidiform mole and missed abortion.

Swelling of Leg

- Very often, usually in later weeks of pregnancy there may be swelling of legs, sometimes associated with swelling of other parts of the body. The following important points are to be noted:
  - Duration of swelling
  - The exact site of swelling
  - Whether swelling is noticed around the face on getting up from bed in the morning
  - Relation with amount of urinary output.

Difficulty in Respiration

Patients may have difficulty in respiration during the later part of pregnancy. The growing uterus pushes up from below and leads to respiratory embarrassment. Usually, this difficulty increases while lying on bed.

Muscle Cramp

Muscle cramp particularly of lower limbs is common during pregnancy. There is no actual pain but patients complain of some pulling sensation.

Back Pain

Back pain of varied intensity is common during pregnancy. Sometimes the pain may radiate down to one or both lower limbs. Back pain may start at any period of pregnancy.

Menstrual History

A detailed menstrual history starting from menarche should be noted.

Age at Menarche

The exact age of menarche should be noted. In case it is difficult to find out the exact date and approximated date should be taken.

Cycle

Menstrual cycle is the interval between two menstrual periods. For most of the women the cycle is 28 days. The range is from 21–35 days. The first day of the bleeding period is taken as the first day of the cycle. The exact nature of the cycle is important to calculate the expected date of delivery. So any variation of the cycle should be noted with care. If the cycle is irregular the exact pattern should be noted. Sometimes irregular cycle may be followed by one or two regular cycles immediately before conception. Special attention should be paid to the nature of last menstrual cycle.

Duration of Bleeding Phase

Duration of bleeding phase may vary from 3–10 days in general, but in most women it is 3–5 days. The first day of bleeding is taken as the first day of the cycle, though the bleeding on the first day may be less than on the 2nd or the 3rd day. In some women there may be spotting or bleeding for a short duration on completion of the first or the second month of conception. Bleeding on completion of the first month may be confused as last menstrual period. So the interval after which bleeding occurs, the amount of bleeding and the association of other symptoms such as pain should be asked and noted clearly.

Flow

Menstrual flow also varies from individual to individual. Usually heavy flow or flow associated with passage of clot may indicate some gynecological condition prior to conception. Scanty flow only during the last cycle may help to determine the last menstrual period.

Pain

Mild pain in lower abdomen or back is common accompaniment of ovulatory cycle. Excessive pain during menstruation in a parous woman indicates presence of associated gynecological condition.

Calculation of Expected Date of Delivery

The average length of human gestation is 280 days, calculated from the first day of the last menstrual period. The expected date of delivery (EDD) or expected date of confinement (EDC) is calculated by addition of nine calendar months and 7 days to the first day of the last menstrual period. Alternatively it can be calculated by addition of 7 days to the first day of last menstrual period and counting back three calendar months. So the date of last menstrual period (LMP) should be asked and noted clearly. It must be remembered that calculation of EDD by this method is reliable only when the previous menstrual cycles are regular. This point is important in the diagnosis of post-dated pregnancy.

Many women do not remember the date of the last menstrual period. In that case doctor should try to find out the approximate date by asking some leading questions in relation to some religious festival like Puja, Phakua, Moharam, etc. Some women, the Mohammedan women in particular gives menstrual history in relation to the moon. It is desirable that the doctor should have a fair knowledge of the different calendars in use in a particular region.

Quickening

Another way to find out the approximate duration of gestation is to ask about quickening. Quickening is the first sensation of fetal movement felt by the pregnant women. A primigravida women feels the movement first at about 20 weeks and an experienced multigravid women feels it earlier at about 18 weeks of pregnancy. But the problem is, very often they forget the exact date of quickening or do not take notice of it.

Past Medical History

Pregnancy is a physiologic state with profound alteration in the health status. Thus a physiologic state with further alteration may rapidly deteriorate into a pathologic one. Hence the state of pregnancy may adversely affect a pre-existing medical or surgical condition, which in turn may influence the course and outcome of the present pregnancy. Detailed history of medical conditions from childhood onwards should be noted carefully. The following are the conditions which need special attention.

Rheumatic Fever and Heart Disease

Every patient should be asked about rheumatic fever with shifting joint pain in early childhood. Majority of heart disease in our country are sequel of rheumatic fever. In case of established heart disease the following points should be noted:

- Since when she is suffering
- Whether she had heart failure previously or heart failure during previous pregnancy and labor
- Whether she had difficulty in breathing and if so, whether it was during rest or exertion
- History of edema of leg and face
- Whether she consulted a doctor or not. History of use drug and how long she is taking it.

If the patient had cardiac surgery we should know:

- The nature of the disease
- The nature of operation done
- The date of operation
- Presence of symptoms.

Diabetes Mellitus

- History of diabetes mellitus prior to pregnancy
- Duration of disease
- Drug used
- History of gestational diabetes in last pregnancy, drug used, perinatal outcome, birth weight of the baby and any other associated complication.

Hypertension

- History of hypertension in nonpregnant state
- In hypertensive woman – duration of hypertension
- Drug used
- Complications, if any
- Perinatal outcome of previous pregnancy, if any.

Kidney Diseases

History of kidney diseases particularly acute nephritis in childhood, chronic nephritis, pyelitis and pyelonephritis should be asked. In case a patient gives positive history of kidney disease a detailed history should be taken. History of operation on kidney should be asked and noted. History of operation on ureter and urinary bladder, if any, should also be noted.

Pulmonary Tuberculosis

In our country pulmonary tuberculosis is still very common and pregnancy in such a woman is not uncommon. In patients with pulmonary tuberculosis the baby in neonatal period may be infected. So, in a patient with positive history of pulmonary tuberculosis detailed information regarding duration of the disease and drug used should be noted.

Venereal Disease

Venereal disease particularly syphilis infects the baby even in utero. In suspected cases, history of exposure should be taken and in diagnosed cases one should enquire whether treatment was completed or not.

Surgical History

Surgery on heart, lung and kidney may modify the management of subsequent pregnancy and labor. Similarly past operation on uterus, lower genital tract influence the line of management of patient, particularly the management of labor.

Past Gynecological History

The important past gynecological history includes history of pelvic infection following delivery or abortion, abnormal vaginal discharge and/or irregular menstrual pattern. History of tuberculosis anywhere and in pelvis particularly should be asked for. Operation on uterus which need special mention are dilatation and curettage, myomectomy, utriculoplasty (plastic repair of the uterus), amputation of cervix. Other operative procedures which should be noted are pelvic floor repair, repair of complete perineal tear, successful repair of vesicovaginal fistula, etc.

History of Contraceptive

Enquiry should be made of use of contraceptive, if any. The type and duration of use should be noted. If the contraceptive is discontinued the cause of discontinuation should be enquired. Did she have any problem during the use of contraceptive.

Personal History

Through personal history an attempt is made to ascertain the personality of the patient, her food habit, home condition, relation with other family members and her attitude towards the present pregnancy. Till recently most of our woman folk were housewives and lived in a large joint family, where responsibilities were shared almost equally by other family members. But with the passage of time and with changed social and economic orders some of them particularly in urban areas have taken up jobs outside their home.

❐ GYNECOLOGY

Presenting Symptoms

Pain Abdomen

In gynecology patient comes for consultation with some definite complaints. These should be noted in chronological order. Some specific leading questions needed to complete the details of these symptoms are described.

Pain: Pain is the most common complaint in gynecological clinic. Pain is one of the presenting symptoms in many gynecological conditions or it may be the only symptom. During history taking the following points are taken into accounts.

Onset of pain is characteristic in certain condition. Onset may be acute or insidious. Sudden acute pain is characteristic of disturbed ectopic pregnancy, abortion, acute appendicitis, torsion of pelvic tumor and renal colic etc. Chronic pain is usually insidious in nature as in chronic pelvic inflammatory disease, endometriosis, etc.

Exact location of pain is important as it may indicate the organ of origin of pain. Enquiry should be made in which quadrant of abdomen pain starts. To start with pain may be slight and localized but later on may spread to whole abdomen with increasing intensity. Sometimes patient may complain of pain in vulva or perineum only. Next point to ask is the nature of the pain. Colicky pain is due to spasm of a hollow viscus whereas dull acting pain is due to irritation of abdomen by some irritating fluid inside. Colicky or spasmodic pain in lower abdomen is usually of uterine or bowel origin.

To know the duration of pain she should be asked since when she is having pain. Is it continuous or intermittent in nature. If intermittent how long it continues in one episode. Does it radiate to other places like back or towards the thighs.

Relation with menstruation: Enquiry should be made about relation of pain with menstruation. Whether pain starts before, during or after menstruation. Sometimes initially pain is felt cyclically in relation to menstruation but subsequently it may be felt throughout the cycle with increase in intensity as in cases of endometriosis. In spasmodic dysmenorrhoea pain starts with onset of bleeding and may last for few hours to 1–2 days. While in chocolate cyst of ovary, in early stage, when there is pain, it starts after onset of bleeding. Secondary dysmenorrhea usually starts 4–5 days before onset of menstruation and lasts for few days. Another example of cyclical pain is ovulation pain or Mittelschmerz pain. It is a midcycle pain, usually mild to moderate in intensity and self-limiting. Usually it is restricted to one side of the pelvis. Pain during coitus or dyspareunia should be enquired in cases of chronic pain.

Relation with gastrointestinal system: Patient may come to gynecologist with lower abdominal pain of gastrointestinal origin alone or gynecological condition with associated gastrointestinal problem. Pain may be associated with constipation or periodic loose motion, nausea and/or vomiting. Irritable bowel syndrome may cause chronic pelvic pain. Pain is acute and severe in acute appendicitis and in acute diverticulitis.

Relation with urinary system: Acute urinary infection may cause acute and severe pain in lower abdomen. Pain may be aggravated during urination. Sometimes dull aching suprapubic pain may be there which is relived by urination. Ureteric colic is usually acute and colicky in nature.

Other complaints of the patients includes excessive white discharge per vagina, abnormalities of menstruation, something coming out per vagina, etc. Another important cause for gynecological consultation is inability to conceive. These are discussed in detail later.

chapter

8 Physical Examination

The examination room should be well-ventilated with good light, preferably natural light. There should be special arrangement of light to inspect the vagina and cervix. The room should be adequately covered. Equipments for complete examination should be available inside the room. These include:

- Height and weight machine or measuring tape attached to wall
- Weighing machine
- Blood pressure instrument, stethoscope
- Fetal stethoscope, measuring tape
- Sterilized surgical gloves
- Double bladed vaginal speculum
- Anterior vaginal wall retractor
- Swab folding forceps.

The additional equipments necessary for gynecological examination of a patient are:

- Cusco's speculum
- Punch biopsy forceps
- Gauge, pad
- Swab stick in sterile tube
- Glass slide, cover slide
- Few sterile vials
- Formaline, normal saline
- Kopline's jar with preservative.

A female attendant should be present at the time of examination.

Pregnancy is not a diseased condition, but a physiological process with changes in physical state. It is very difficult to demonstrate the degree of changes beyond which it turns to be pathological. So majority of the antenatal cases are healthy woman without any disease. Keeping this point in mind antenatal cases are examined and findings are noted. As gynecology deals with diseases of the female genital tract the doctor should be careful in interpretation of the examination findings. Findings should be correlated with the presenting complaints. Basically methods of examination are same as followed in medical and surgical units, which include inspection, palpation, percussion and auscultation. Though the woman may not have any complaint she should be examined as a whole. All the systems should be examined carefully, specially on her first visit. For example, valvular heart disease may remain asymptomatic and might be missed which may turn to be serious at a later period of pregnancy or during labor.

The first step in physical examination is observation of the patient, to assess the general appearance and attitude. Ideally observation should start as the patient enters the consultation room.

❒ GENERAL APPEARANCE

Assessment of general appearance is made quickly – whether the patient is ill or healthy, her nutritional status, presence of any sign of distress are noted. This is an important step as a severely ill patient may need immediate treatment. A case of severe pre-eclampsia or impending eclampsia may not have any complaint but she needs immediate treatment.

❒ ATTITUDE

Attitude of the patient is important in certain conditions such as acute abdomen. In colicky pain the patient is restless, but in pain due to peritonitis she remains still.

❒ GAIT

Gait of the patient is observed when she walks. Different abnormal gaits may influence the shape and hence the capacity of the pelvis.

❒ NUTRITION

Generally it is sufficient to note whether the patient is lean or fat. Under-nutrition is a common problem of the women in developing countries. Particular deficiency factors should be searched for and noted. Obesity is of particular importance in certain gynecological condition.

❒ HEIGHT AND WEIGHT

Height and weight of the patient are recorded. The importance of recording height is that from height one can assume the capacity of the bony pelvis. A woman with short stature (5 feet or less) is likely to have a small pelvis.

To record weight throughout pregnancy is a time honoured procedure. Rate of weight gain during different period of pregnancy is different and varies from individual to individual. Excessive weight gain during later months of pregnancy is due to excessive water accumulation (occult or evident) and is a warning sign of pre-eclampsia. The average total gain in weight during pregnancy is about 11 kg which may vary between 6 kg and 15 kg. The increase should not be more than 13 kg. During the first trimester total gain is about 1 kg. only. Thereafter, the increase should be at the rate of 0.5 kg in one week and a gain of 0.7 kg in one week is regarded as abnormal. Though excessive weight gain is not a reliable sign of impending pre-eclampsia it is sufficiently valuable to record patient's weight in every antenatal visit. In an ICMR study conducted in different centers of India the average maternal weight at 20 weeks of gestation was found to be 49.0 kg and an increase to 54.8 kg at 36 weeks, giving an overall gain of 0.36 kg per week. Further, it was observed that the overall weight gain in those mothers who delivered low birth weight babies was 3.5–4 kg less than those who had babies of normal birth weight.

❐ PULSE

The arterial pulse during pregnancy is of large volume while in cachectic and anemic women the pulse might be thready. Pulse should be counted for full one minute. The resting pulse rate increases during pregnancy by about 10–15 beats per minute. Cardiac arrhythmia like ectopic beat may occur in some normal pregnant women without evidence of heart disease.

Blood Pressure

Blood pressure should be measured in the antenatal check-up and subsequently in each visit. Pre-pregnancy blood pressure if available or blood pressure taken at early pregnancy is taken as baseline pressure for subsequent evaluation. In clinical practice blood pressure is measured with sphygmomanometer. The pressure is taken with the patient either recumbent or sitting position with the upper arm at the level with the heart. In supine position the gravid uterus often interferes with venous return from the lower part of the body and therefore blood pressure recorded in that position may be erroneous. So, the student should be familiar with the correct procedure. The patient should be asked to lie on right side with 30 degree of tilt towards the observer. In this position the upper arm remains at the level of the heart. She should be comfortable at this position. The sphygmomanometer cuff is applied over inside of upper arm with connecting tubes to sphygmomanometer pointing head wards. The lower margin of the cuff should be 2 cm above the antecubital fossa. The cuff should be applied evenly and firmly but not tightly. Feeling of brachial artery pulse in the antecubital fossa stethoscope is placed directly over it and held in place. Inflate the cuff to 20–30 mm of Hg above the point at which Korotkoff sounds disappear. The mercury column is allowed to fall steadily at 2–3 mm per second. The systolic pressure is taken at the point at which the tapping Korotkoff sound first becomes audible for two consecutive beats (Korotkoff Phase-I). The second record is taken where the sound first becomes muffled (Korotkoff Phase -IV). This point marks the diastolic pressure. Sometimes, the second point is not precise, the clear sound changing only imperceptible to muffle sound. If no clear point of muffling is noticed the point of disappearance of Korotkoff sound (Korotkoff Phase-V) is to be taken. Then the air is let down completely. If needed measurement should be repeated, but before the next measurement the cuff should be completely deflated and mercury column should be at O level. It should be remembered that in good number of women both normal and hypertensive, blood pressure falls during the second trimester and rise again in third trimester and may reach the pre-pregnancy level at term.

Pallor

Pallor means paleness and pallor is due to anemia. Anemia is a condition of qualitative reduction in hemoglobin concentration of blood. In under-developed countries anemia is the number one cause of maternal death. So every effort should be made to detect anemia early and to try to treat adequately. Color of the mucus membrane of mouth and conjunctive gives better indication of pallor. Color of the skin is most misleading. Both the lower lids of the eyes are gently pulled downwards while the patient is asked to look upwards and the conjunctive are examined for color. The fallacies are if the patient is suffering from conjunctivitis or if she is emotionally upset the color of conjunctive is changed. The other sites of importance are tongue, nail bed and palmer creases.

Jaundice

Jaundice is best examined in the sclera. The sclera becomes yellowish. The upper lids of eyes ares gently pulled upwards while the patient is asked to look downwards. Yellow discolorations of the under surface of the tongue also gives a good indication of jaundice.

Teeth and Gum

An infected tooth is the source of infection. A careful search should be made to detect such tooth. Gum also should be examined in every patient.

Neck Veins

Presence of enlarged and/or pulsating neck veins should be noted, as the condition indicates decompensated condition of the heart.

Edema

Edema or swelling of tissue is caused by accumulation of excessive fluid in the subcutaneous space. Edema of legs is common condition during pregnancy. Due to different conditions legs become edematous. Though leg edema is common during pregnancy there may be edema of abdominal wall, face and hand also. Severity of edema is indicated as 1+ , 2+, 3+ and 4+.

1+ : edema confined below the knee.

2+ : edema extends upward involving the whole of lower limbs.

3+ : Leg edema with edema of anterior abdominal wall.

4+ : Generalized edema.

Previously edema was thought to be an important symptom of pre-ecampsia. But in about half of the primigravida women leg edema may be present at later weeks of pregnancy without any complication. But severe edema or rapidly developing edema is significant and to be viewed with caution. It is almost always common with anemia and general malnutrition.

Besides swelling of legs, patient may give history of tightening of ring or tightening of shoes. To elicit edema gently pressure is applied over the shin of the tibia for about 20 seconds, and lifting the fingers note for any depression. In a bed-ridden patient pressure should be applied over the back of the sacrum as it is the most dependant part in them.

Varicose Veins

Vericose vein in the lower limb is a distressing condition for some pregnant women. For varicose vein the patient should be examined in standing position. Tendelenberg's test may be done to assess the efficiency of the valves of the saphenous vein.

❒ SYSTEMIC EXAMINATION

The woman should be examined thoroughly in her first visit to obtain certain baseline information regarding her health status. These informations help the clinician to evaluate any deviation from normalcy. It should be remembered that pregnancy itself causes certain deviation from normal non-pregnant state due to its profound effect on various systems of the body. These anatomical and physiological changes will be discussed briefly here. These physiological changes may cause some discomfort or symptoms which are temporary and usually need no treatment.

The methods of examination of various systems of the body are same as in other branches of medicine. So, only the alterations caused by pregnancy will be dealt here.

Cardiovascular System

During pregnancy due to the growing uterus the diaphragm is elevated progressively. As a result the heart is displaced to the left and upwards with slight axial rotation. Along with these changes there are some alteration in the heart sound also. There are an exaggerated splitting of the first heart sound and a loud third sound. A systolic murmur is often present and a soft diastolic murmur may also be present in few women.

Mammary Murmur

A continuous murmur from the mammary artery may be heard over the 2nd and 3rd intercostals spaces mostly on the left side. The intensity can be varied by the pressure exerted with the stethoscope on the chest wall. The murmur continues during the first few weeks of lactation and generally disappears towards the end of the second month after delivery.

Cardiac Output

Cardiac output at rest increases during pregnancy. It increases during the end of the first trimester and remains elevated during the rest of the period of pregnancy. This increase is much higher in lateral recumbent position as the growing uterus pressing over the inferior vena cava reduces venous return to the heart.

Respiratory System

In pregnancy the diaphragm is raised without disturbing its movements during respiration. The circumference of the thoracic cage increases and the subcostal angle widens. Functionally also some changes take place. Vital capacity remains unaltered but there is increase in tidal volume (the amount of air exchanged at each breath while at rest) and the respiratory rate. The pregnant woman breathes more deeply and more rapidly at rest. Increased awareness of a desire to breath is common. This may be interpreted as dyspnea. Thus it appears that pregnancy does not impair pulmonary function.

Gastrointestinal System

Along with diminution in tone and motility of smooth muscles there is decreased tone and motility of the gastrointestinal tract also. Gastric emptying time is prolonged. Sphincters are relaxed. As a result reflux of gastric juice into the esophagus causes heart burn. And constipation is very common among pregnant women. Increased venous pressure may cause hemorrhoids in many cases. Important among the anatomical changes is displacement of the vermiform appendix upwards and laterally as the uterus enlarges.

Examination of Breast and Nipple

Breast and nipple should be examined during the antenatal period. Normally nipple is cylindrical and projects well beyond the surface of the breast.

In some cases nipples may be depressed or it may be inverted. In such cases attempts should be made with fingers to draw it out.

Abdominal Examination

Complete examination of the alimentary system should be carried out at the first visit. This includes examination of the gastrointestinal tract, liver and spleen. Attempts should be made to exclude, any palpable condition of kidney or the urinary bladder. During the first trimester as the uterus remains as a pelvic organ there is no difficulty in palpating the abdominal viscera. During the later part of pregnancy the growing uterus displaces the intestines laterally and makes it difficult to properly palpate the other organs.

❐ OBSTETRIC EXAMINATION

Before discussing details of obstetric examination certain terms should be known.

Lie: Lie of the fetus means relation of the long axis of the fetus to the long axis of the uterus. The lie may be longitudinal, transverse or oblique.

Presentation

The part of the fetus which is in relation to the cervix is the presenting part. The presenting part can be felt through the cervix on vaginal examination. The presenting part determines the presentation. When the head occupies the lower pole of the uterus there may be three different presentations. If the head is fully flexed so that the chin is in contact with the thorax, the presentation is vertex: if the head is fully extended, the presentation is face and if midway between flexion and extension the presentation is brow. When the breech occupies the lower part of the uterus the presentation is breech. And when the fetus lies transversely the shoulder is the presenting part.

Position

Position is the relation of a given part of the fetus to the maternal pelvis. A fix point, selected in each presentation is called denominator. In vertex presentation the point is occiput and in face presentation the point is the mentum. The relation of denominator to the different quadrant of the pelvis is known as position. In vertex presentation if the occiput is on the left side and anterior the position is left occipito-anterior (LOA).

Attitude

The relation of different parts of the fetus to each other is known as attitude. If the back, the head and the limbs are flexed the attitude is of flexion, if extended the attitude is extension. Usually at term the fetus forms an ovoid mass with flexion attitude. The back is markedly flexed, head is flexed so that the chin is almost in contact with the thorax, the thighs are bent up towards the abdomen and the knees are bent. Arms and forearms are also flexed and crossed over the thorax. This fetal ovoid is accommodated well inside the uterine cavity.

Abdominal Examination

The patient is asked to evacuate the bladder before examination. She should lie on her back on examination table and abdomen is fully exposed. The shoulder should be slightly raised and knees bent slightly.

Inspection

During early pregnancy there is not much change in abdominal wall. One should note whether there is any scar or any skin disease.

After 20 weeks of pregnancy enlargement of the lower half of the abdomen is noticeable. At the same time there is appearance of reddish, slightly depressed streak in the skin of the lower abdomen. These are called stria gravidarum. Stria gravidarum may develop over the breast and over the thighs also. In some women the midline skin of the abdomen becomes pigmented with brownish-black color. This is known as linea nigra. Besides skin condition the uterine swelling is noted, whether it is widely enlarged, pyriform or spherical in shape. In transverse lie the uterus appears to be wider than usual. Sometimes during later part of pregnancy fetal movement can be seen through the abdominal wall.

Palpation

During the first trimester the uterus remains as a pelvic organ and cannot be felt abdominally. It can be felt abdominally at 12 weeks of gestation. With thin abdominal wall the uterus can be felt after 10 weeks.

Upto 28 weeks of pregnancy fetal lie, presentation and position are not important, only the following few points are noted.

Braxton Hicks Contraction

During pregnancy, uterus undergoes spontaneous contraction which can be felt on placing the hand over the uterus. These irregular and painless contractions are known as Braxton-Hicks contractions.

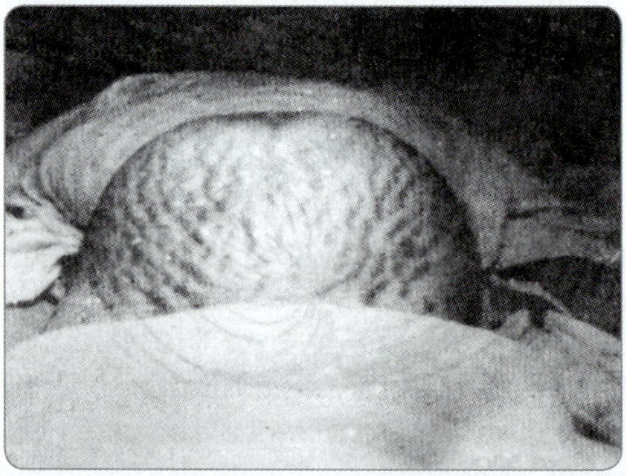

Fig. 1: Sria gravidarum

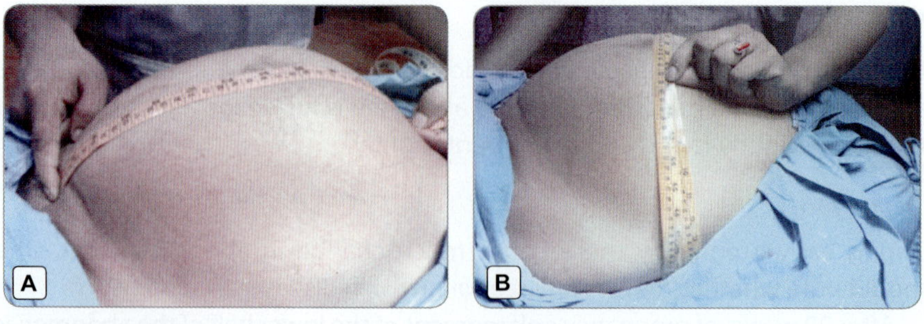

Figs 2A and B: Measurement of symphysis—fundal height and Girth of the abdomen

Palpation of Fetal Parts

On gentle palpation of the uterus fetal parts can be felt with active fetal movement.

External Ballotment

Around 20 weeks of pregnancy the fetus is small in relation to the amount of liquor amnii present. So a sudden pressure exerted on one side of the uterus displaces the fetus and then rebound to its original position and a tap is felt by the examining fingers. This is however difficult to elicit in obese patient.

During the third trimester special attention is paid to detect the lie, presentation, and position of the fetus in uterus. The following points are noted carefully.

Height of the fundus or fundal height: Along with the gradual increase in the size of the uterus the fundal height increases. Upto 12 weeks of pregnancy the uterus remains almost globular, thereafter upto 36 weeks the enlargement is more longitudinal and the shape of the uterus is elliptical. After 36 weeks the uterus again becomes more or less globular. Accordingly the fundal height changes. From the height of the fundus approximate duration of pregnancy can be ascertained. Three different landmarks are taken to express fundal height in relation to different periods of gestation. Fundus is palpable above the symphysis pubis at 12 weeks of pregnancy, just above the umbilicus at 24th week and near the xiphoid cartilage at 36 weeks of pregnancy. The part

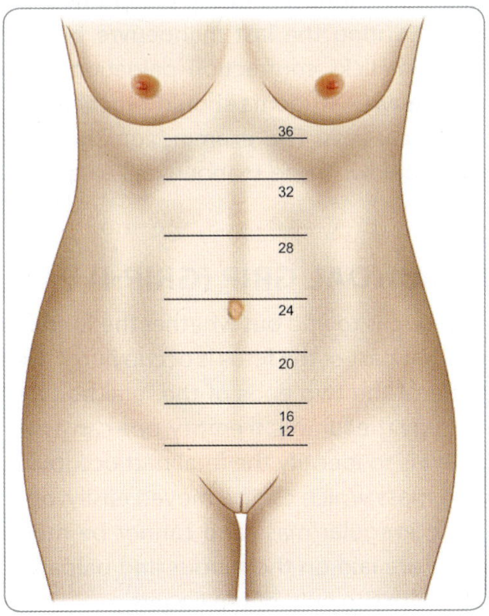

Fig. 3: Height of the fundus of the uterus at different weeks of pregnancy

between symphysis pubis and umbilicus is again divided into two equal parts as 16th and 20th week. And the part between umbilicus and xiphoid cartilage is divided into 28th and 32nd week of pregnancy. After 36 weeks the fundus of the uterus drops by about 2–3 inches and the shape of the uterus becomes more or less globular.

The examiner stands on the right side of the patient facing towards the abdomen. The upper border of the left hand is placed few centimeters above the abdominal bulge and gradually brought down to feel the top of the fundus. Keeping the hand there, duration of pregnancy in weeks is assessed as described earlier. It is a good habit to measure the fundal height from the upper border of the symphysis pubis with a measuring tape calibrated in centimeter. Along with the fundal height, circumference/girth of the abdomen at the level of the umbilicus should be measured at each visit and noted for future reference (Fig. 2A and B). It is demonstrated that between 18th and 30th week of gestation the fundal height in centimeters equals the gestational age in weeks. Fundal height in cm along with abdominal circumference can give an idea of fetal growth in utero.

Diagnosis of presentation and position of the fetus: Abdominal palpation should be performed systematically for accurate diagnosis. There are four manoeuvres for abdominal palpation which should be carried out gently. In no case jerky movement should be applied. It should be remembered that lower part of the uterus is usually tender and only gentle pressure should be applied so that the patient does not resist. During the first three manoeuvers the examiner stands on the right side of the patient near the examining table facing the patient and during the last manoeuvre he faces the feet of the patient. During Braxton-Hicks contraction palpation is not done. To attain the skill in these manoeuvres students should practice it during their clinical attachments in obstetric wards. The examination should be systematic and should be followed as below. These manoeuvres or grips were described by Leopold.

❐ FIRST GRIP: FUNDAL GRIP (GRIP-I)

The idea of the fundal grip is to find out whether the fundus of the uterus is full or empty, and if full, what part of the fetus is occupying it. Generally as the fetus lies longitudinally one of the two ends of the fetal body, i.e. the head or the buttocks (breech) occupy the fundus. If empty, one can assume that the fetus is lying transversely. Next is to identify the fetal part occupying the fundus. Fetal head is globular, hard mass which can be moved easily, on the other hand the breech is a bulky, soft, irregular mass and cannot be moved easily. Both the palms of the examiner are laid on the fundus and palpation of the fetal parts are carried out gently with the pulp of the fingers.

❒ SECOND GRIP: LATERAL GRIP (GRIP-II)

Lateral grip is carried out to identify on which side the back lies. The back of the fetus is represented by a uniformly resistant, smooth surface. On the opposite side are knob- like structures representing the fetal limbs. The examiner places both his hands on the sides of the abdomen. From one side a gentle pressure is applied and palpation is carried on the opposite side. The same procedure is repeated on the other side also. Sometimes, particularly in primigravida cases with strong anterior abdominal wall and in obese patient it may be difficult to recognize the knob-like structures representing the fetal limbs. The back is not felt if it lies directly posteriorly, then of course the fetal limbs are easily felt on both sides of the mid line. The next point is to determine the position of the back, whether it is directed **anteriorly,** laterally or posteriorly.

❒ THIRD GRIP: PAWLIK'S GRIP (GRIP-III)

With this manoeuvre the part of the fetus occupying the lower pole of the uterus is ascertained. Presentation can be determined and whether the presenting part is engaged or not can also be known. The **ulner** border of the right hand is placed over the symphysis pubis with the thumb on one side and the four fingers on other. The lower part of the maternal abdomen is gently grasped. The presenting part is felt and determined whether it is head or breech. If the presenting part is not engaged or not **fixed** at the brim it can be moved from side to side. In case of

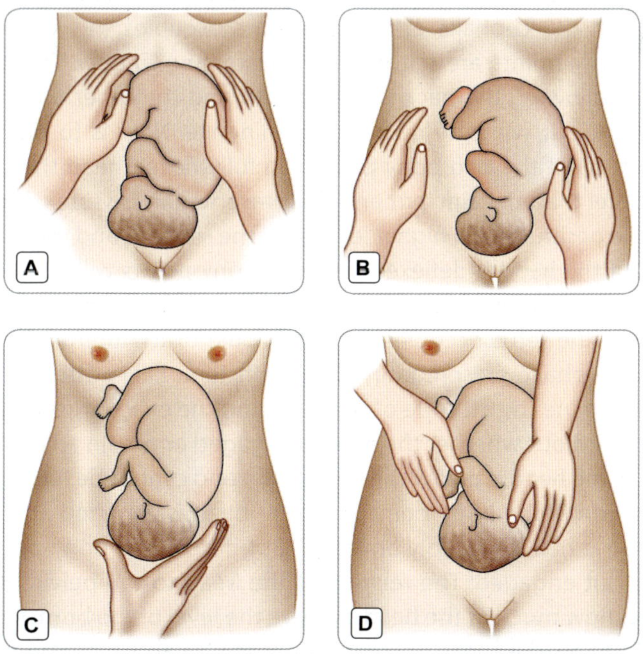

Figs 4A to D: (A) Fundal grip; (B) Lateral grip; (C) Pawlik's grip; (D) Pelvic grip

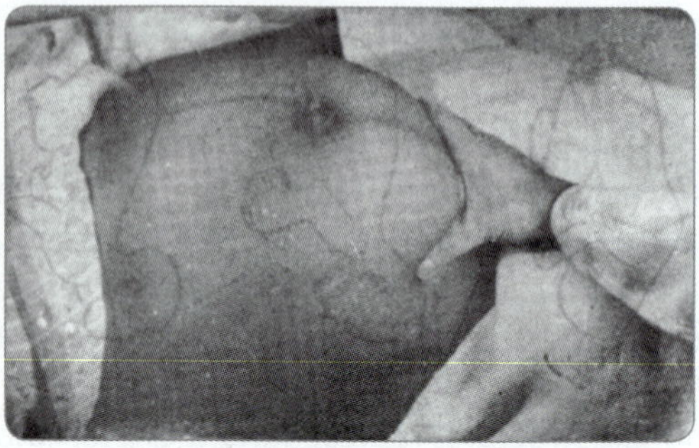

Fig. 5: Pawlik's grip

cephalic presentation, by the position of the cephalic prominence the exact presentation is determined. If the cephalic prominence is on the side of the fetal limbs the head is well-flexed and the presentation is vertex. On the other hand if the cephalic prominence is on the side of the back the head is extended and the presentation is face.

❒ FOURTH GRIP: PELVIC GRIP (GRIP-IV)

This is an important grip as several informations like attitude, presentation and engagement of the presenting part can be obtained. While carrying out this grip the examiner faces towards the feet of the patient. Both the hands are placed on the sides of the lower pole of the fetus and the fingers are gently pressed. When the cephalic end of the fetus occupies the lower pole two prominent bony points are felt with the examining fingers. The bony point which is felt following the back is the **occiput** and the other on the opposite side is the sinciput with the cephalic prominence. Next is to determine the relative position of the two bony points. In fully-flexed head the occiput lies at a lower level than the sinciput and the presentation is vertex. If the head is extended the occiput is at a higher level than the sinciput and the presentation is face. And if the head is deflexed both the bony points will be at same level and the presentation is brow. It should be remembered that in most of the cases head of the fetus occupies the lower pole of the uterus. And a simple diagnosis of cephalic presentation is not sufficient. Every attempt should be made to determine the attitude of the head and the exact presentation.

Next is to find out whether the head is engaged or not. In an engaged head major part of the head is below the pelvic brim and cannot be felt abdominally. On examination if one bony point is felt the head is engaged and if no bony point is felt the head is deeply engaged. But if both the bony points are felt the head is not engaged. The relation of the head to the pelvic brim can be described as how much of the head is above the level of the brim. Abdominally the level of the head is measured as number of fifth above the brim. When the head is entirely above the brim it is five-fifths above and a four-fifth above head is just entering the brim. When the head is three-fifths above, the examining hands still go partially round the head. When two-fifths above, the hands **splay** outwards, when one-fifth above only the sinciput can be felt and in zero-fifth no occiput or sinciput is felt.

❐ AUSCULTATION OF FETAL HEART

Fetal heart sound is auscultated to know the condition of the fetus. It is best auscultated with fetal stethoscope (fetoscope). The widest end is pressed over the back of the fetus and the heart sound is auscultated. Fetal heart sound is best heard over the left scapular region, so area of maximum intensity varies according to the position of the back. A search should be made moving the fetoscope to locate the area of maximum intensity of the sound. Usually the area of maximum intensity lies over an imaginary line joining the anterior superior **iliac** spine and the umbilicus. In breech presentation this level is higher. In posterior position heart sound can be heard over the chest of the fetus at the side of the midline. In face presentation also fetal heart sound is heard through the chest of the fetus.

Immediately after locating the area of maximum intensity the examiner should feel the radial pulse of the mother. Fetal heart sound does not coincide with the maternal pulse. This helps the examiner to differentiate a uterine soufflé from fetal heart sound.

Rate of the fetal heart sound is counted for full two minutes. Normally fetal heart sound should be between 120–160 beats per minute. A rate below 120 beats per minute is called fetal bradycardia and above 160 beats per minute is called fetal tachycardia. Both these indicate fetal jeopardy. Another important factor is rhythm of the fetal heart rate. It should be regular. Irregularity of fetal heart is a grave sign. Around twenty-fourth week of pregnancy and onwards a soft, blowing sound synchronous with the maternal pulse is heard on the lateral aspect of the uterus in the lower part. It is uterine soufflé. It is produced during passage of blood through the enlarged, **tortuous** uterine arteries. When this sound is heard maternal radial pulse should be felt with which it synchronizes.

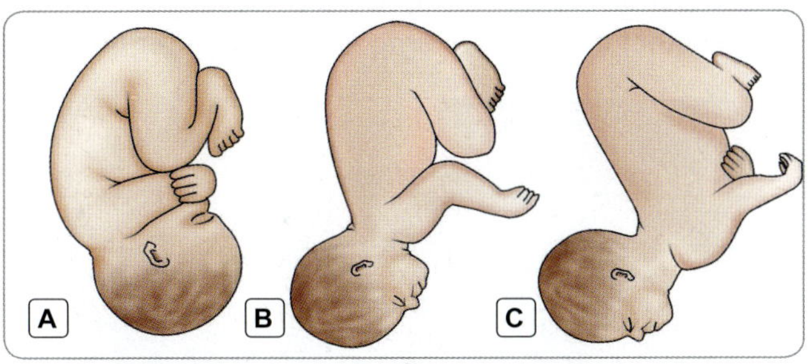

Figs 6A to C: Attitude of the fetal head showing different presentation according to attitude: (A) head is fully flexed – vertex presentation; (B) head is grossly deflexed – brow presentation; (C) head is fully extended – face presentation

❐ VAGINAL EXAMINATION

Vaginal examination is usually restricted during pregnancy, as each vaginal examination may introduce some pathogens into the genital tract. However, there are some specific conditions when vaginal examination is indicated. Vaginal examination when needed should be performed under strict aseptic conditions.

The indications are:

1. For diagnosis of pregnancy in first trimester vaginal examination is necessary. During the first trimester size of the uterus corresponds well with the duration of pregnancy and such a record is very valuable to determine the gestational age if some anomaly arises at later weeks. However, in a patient with history of previous repeated abortion at early weeks, vaginal examination is deferred.
2. In the first visit irrespective of duration of pregnancy a vaginal examination should be done to exclude any pelvic pathology.
3. In primigravida cases vaginal examination is performed after 37th week of pregnancy to assess the capacity of the pelvis.
4. To diagnose labor vaginal examination is mandatory.

In cases of vaginal bleeding during the later weeks of pregnancy vaginal examination should never be done in examination room or in out-patient department. In such a case vaginal examination is only done in operation theater keeping everything ready for caesarean section.

Strict aseptic measures are taken while doing a vaginal examination in a pregnant woman. Hands are properly washed and sterile gloves are put on. Vagina is lubricated with an antiseptic solution. Separating the vulva with the left hand first the index finger of the right hand is introduced gently. At this stage a young primigravida may resist. In that case wait for few moments and gently press over the perineum with the finger inside. Then introduce the middle finger gently. First the cervix is felt, its position, the os and its texture are noted. In early weeks an attempt is made to assess the size of the uterus putting the left hand over the symphysis pubis. Then the sides of the uterus are examined to detect if any extra lump is present. After finishing the entire

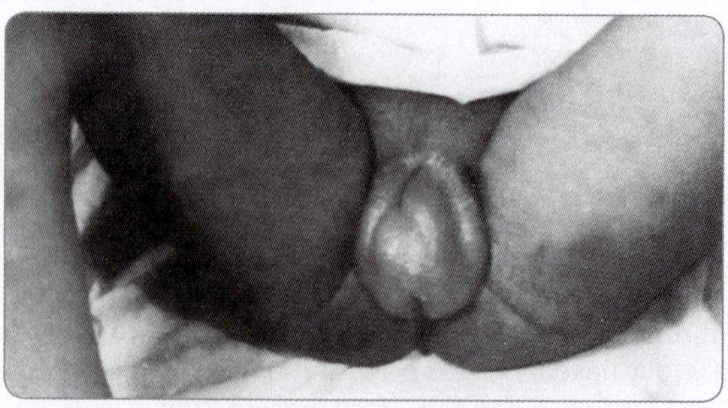

Fig. 7: Gross vulval edema

examination fingers are taken out and the discharge smeared in the examining fingers should be observed and noted if any abnormality is detected.

Follow-up Examination

It is difficult to lay down a fixed schedule of follow-up.

Every patient should be considered individually and called for follow-up examination. However, as a general rule and in an uncomplicated pregnancy during the first six months a pregnant woman should be examined monthly, then every fortnightly upto 36 weeks and then every week till delivery.

In the follow-up examination following points are noted:

Complaints (if any): Complaints of the woman should be noted at each visit and a careful note is kept in the "case note".

General examination: In general examination weight, pulse, blood pressure and edema should be recorded in each visit.

Systemic examination: It also should be carried out if any complaints are there and findings should be noted.

Obstetric examination*:* Upto 26 weeks fetal presentation and position are not important. So the examination is confined to measuring the fundal height and auscultation of the fetal heart sound. Thereafter, of course, a thorough examination is carried out to detect the height of the fundus, fetal presentation, position and fetal heart sound.

Ripe Cervix

The cervix is said to be ripe when it is short, soft and slightly dilated. The internal os is also dilated and admits tip of a finger. It is a prelabor preparation of the cervix for actual onset of labor. But sometimes the cervix may remain in this state for days together. A ripe cervix is ideal, though the cervix may remain at any state even before labor.

Bishop Score

Bishop score indicates the state of the cervix. Few features of the cervix itself, its relation with the presenting part besides dilatation and effacement are considered and each feature is given a score. The summation of the score gives an overall idea of the cervical maturity and particularly of its possible response to induction of labor.

Score	0	1	2	3
Dilatation (cm)	0	1–2	3–4	5–6
Effacement %	0–30	40–50	60–70	80+
Station (cm) above spine	–3	–2	–1, 0	(cm) below +1, +2
Consistency	Firm	Medium	Soft	
Position	Posterior	Mid	Anterior	

If the total score is nine or more induction is likely to be successful.

❒ GYNECOLOGICAL EXAMINATION

Abdominal Examination

Abdominal examination is performed with the patient lying flat on the examination table. Before hand the patient is asked to pass urine so that the urinary bladder remains empty. It is preferable to have an empty rectum too. While lying flat on the table knees are slightly flexed so that abdominal muscles are relaxed. The abdomen should be fully exposed. Examination is performed systematically.

During examination of the patient relaxation of the abdominal wall is very important. Lying flat on the examination table legs are slightly flexed. Sometimes muscle guard due to inflammation also makes abdominal wall taut. Some women cannot relax the abdomen out of fear or apprehension. In such situation she is asked to take deep breath and the examiner should try to divert the attention of the women with conversation.

Inspection

On inspection size, shape of the abdomen, presence of swelling on any quadrant of the abdomen, skin condition, presence of scar, presence of linea nigra or presence of pigmentation are noted. It is useful to note movement of the abdominal wall with respiration. Sometimes with huge abdominal swelling the umbilicus may be everted.

Palpation

Palpation of the abdomen should be very gentle, particularly in patients with acute abdominal pain. Hand should be warm. During cold weather it is sufficient to rub both palms against each other to make it warm. Palpation is done with flat of the hands. Use of finger tips may hurt the patient. If the patient gives history of pain abdomen she is asked to locate the area of pain with her finger. As a rule palpation should be started from an area away from the area of origin of pain and gradually go near that area to elicit tenderness. After the tender area is found the point of maximum tenderness is searched which will help to

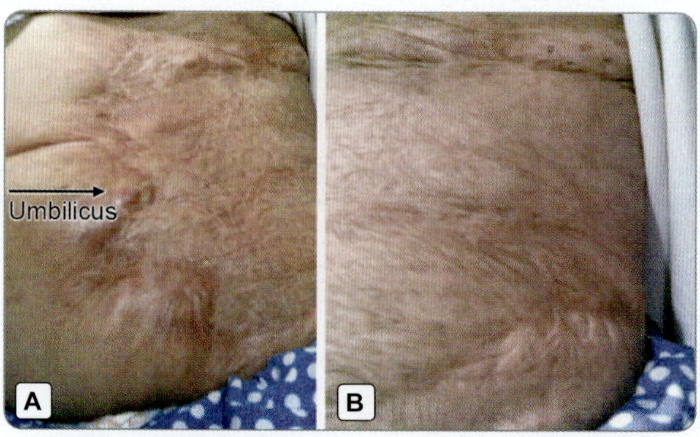

Figs 8A and B: Scar of anterior abdominal wall

assume the organ of origin of pain. Sometimes a patient may not be able to pin pointedly locate the area of pain, but vaguely moves her hand over an area of the abdomen. In that case also palpation is started away from that area and the area of tenderness is to be elicited. After superficial palpation deep palpation is carried out to confirm the findings of superficial palpation.

When a lump is detected in lower abdomen its size, shape, position, mobility and consistency are determined. Presence of fluid in peritoneal cavity can be determined by palpation. Presence of fluid can also be detected by fluid thrill from one side of the abdomen to the other. When the amount of fluid is less it can be demonstrated by shifting dullness. If fluid is detected in the peritoneal cavity attempt should be made to find out presence of solid tumor. This is done by sudden dipping down of the fingers deep into the abdomen.

To exclude pregnancy in a cystic midline suprapubic swelling two important signs associated with pregnancy Braxton-Hicks contraction and ballotment are elicited.

Percussion

The next step is percussion. With the help of percussion one can know whether an abdominal lump is dull or tympanatic. A solid lump or a lump filled with fluid is dull on percussion while a tympanatic sound is produced when bowel is there below the abdominal wall or a bowel is situated over the lump. Percussion is important to elicit shifting dullness to determine presence of free fluid in the flanks. It is difficult to differentiate a huge ovarian cyst, filling whole of the abdomen, from ascites. In case of ovarian cyst of this size bowels are pushed towards the flanks, hence flankes are tympanatic on percussion and it is dull on the midline. On the other hand in ascites bowels float on the ascitic fluid, producing tympanatic sound in the midline and dullness over the flanks on percussion.

Auscultation

On auscultation of the abdomen normally only bowel sounds are heard. Bowel sound is absent in cases of intestinal paralysis due to generalized peritonitis and paralytic ileus. Presence of bowel sounds over a lump confirms presence of a loop of bowel, which may be due to adhesion. In pregnant uterus or sometimes in large uterine myoma with hypertrophy of the uterine artery a blowing sound is heard synchronizing with maternal pulse, when the stethoscope is placed over a big vessel. This is uterine soufflé. Fetal heart sound is heard if duration of pregnancy is 24 weeks or more. Fetal heart sound doesn't synchronize with maternal pulse and the rate is more.

Vaginal Examination

Vaginal examination can be carried out in four different positions. Each of these positions has advantages and disadvantages. Care should be taken to minimize exposure of the patient. These position are—lateral, semiprone, dorsal and lithotomy.

Lateral position: In this position the patient turn to her left side and draws up both knees. For the patient it is an easy and comfortable position, avoids undue exposure. A thorough examination can be carried out.

Semiprone or Sim's position: Semiprone position is again known as Sim's position. In this position the patient lies on the left side. Both knees are drawn up , the right one is drawn up slightly more than the left. This allows a good exposure of external genitalia. Vaginal speculum can be introduced easily as such a thorough examination is possible.

Dorsal position: In this position the patient lies on her back with flexed hips and knees. Here exposure is a bit more but allows convenient bimanual examination.

Lithotomy position: This is the position which is usually preferred when examination is done under anesthesia or for any vaginal operation. In this the patient lies on her back, buttocks brought to the edge of the table, hips and knees flexed and legs are slightly abducted . Legs are kept in position with support, fixed at the side of the table.

Method of Examination

There should be sufficient light and the light should be positioned so that vagina and cervix can be seen on speculum examination. Bladder should be empty. The examination should be in a methodical manner and all the parts should be examined with minimum discomfort to the patient.

Vaginal examination is performed usually in dorsal position. Examiner should put on sterile gloves and fingers should be well-lubricated.

First, inspect the skin condition of mons pubis, vulva and perineum to exclude any abnormal swelling, new growth or ulceration. Presence of vaginal discharge should be noted. Then with gloved hands examination is carried out. Initially exploration of vagina and cervix is carried out with the index finger. For bimanual examination it is better to introduce the index and the middle finger provided the vagina is capacious.

With the thumb and index fingers of the left hand labia are separated and vestibule is exposed. Index finger of the right hand is introduced inside the

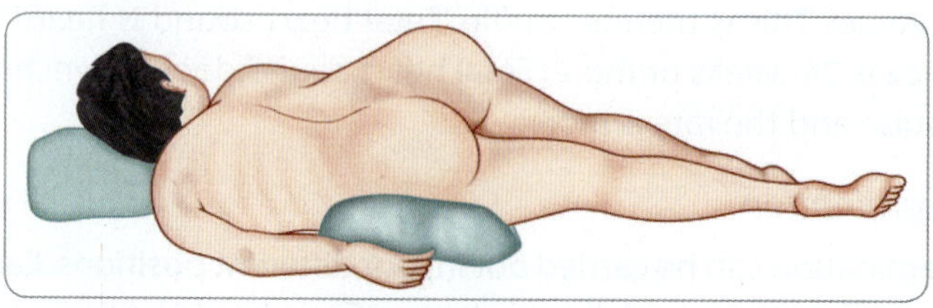

Fig. 9: Sim's position

vagina. Urethra and skenes tubules are massaged from behind forward to see presence or absence of purulent discharge. If purulent discharge is there sample should be taken in sterile swab stick for culture and sensitivity test. The opening of the Bartholin glands are examined. The labia are palpated on either side. Palpation may reveal small solid or cystic swelling. Next is exploration of vagina. The well-lubricated index and middle fingers of the gloved hand are introduced inside the vagina to examine the walls systematically. On exploring the vagina smoothness of the walls, laxity and presence of any cystic lesion or growth are noted. If any lesion is detected its size, shape, consistency and mobility are determined. Next fornices are explored from one side to the other. Fornices may be shallow or deep. There may be transverse fibrous bands narrowing the area. In case of tumor in the pelvis fornices may bulge or there may be sense of fullness due to collection of fluid or blood in pelvic cavity. Fornices are obliterated at menopause. Next the fingers are directed towards the vaginal portion of the cervix. Usually cervix can be felt easily but sometimes it may be difficult to reach the cervix, when it is placed high up behind the symphysis pubis. Usually a pelvic lump occupying the pouch of Douglas may push the cervix anteriorly and behind the symphysis. Similarly in retroverted gravid uterus also the cervix remains anteriorly and at a higher plane. Sometimes in post-caesarean or post-myomectomy cases uterus may be adherent to the anterior abdominal wall and it is difficult to reach the cervix vaginally. In obese woman also to reach the cervix vaginally is difficult. Length of the vaginal portion is important to note. In deep fornix the length is more. Its direction, size, shapes are noted. In parous women cervix is usually bulky than in nulliparous women, but sometimes it is unduly bulky. Normally the surface is smooth. It may be irregular in presence of growth or rough in erosion. The external os is palpated with the index finger. In parous women external os may admit one finger, but in nulliparous women the cervix may be conical and external os remains closed. While palpating the os one should be very careful, the finger may inadvertently injure a friable growth in the cervix leading to bleeding. Again there may be a polyp, smooth mucus polyp or fibromyomatous polyp. A growth in cervix may be soft or hard, irregular mass. The cervix may be torn on one side or on both sides where the os is wide open.

Speculum Examination

Inspection of the cervix: For inspection of the cervix of the uterus vaginal speculum is used. Different types of vaginal speculum are there, mostly one of the following two types are used:

Sim's speculum or Sim's double bladed speculum—This instrument consists of two concave blades of different size connected by a handle. After introduction inside the vagina the cervix, anterior vaginal wall and vault can be inspected properly. In parous women particularly when there is sagging of the anterior vaginal wall or with cystocele an anterior vaginal wall retractor is needed to retract the vaginal wall. The posterior vaginal wall cannot be inspected after introduction of this speculum. This speculum is commonly used during vaginal operation. The smallest possible speculum which can give a good view of the cervix and vault should be used. In case of nulliparous women and in postmenopausal women with narrow vagina a smaller size speculum should be used.

Cusco's bivalve speculum: This speculum is best suited for examination of the cervix and the vault of vagina. This is a bivalve speculum joined at the base, i.e. the vulval end with a hinge. After introduction inside the vagina the valves can be screwed open and can be kept fixed. No assistant is needed to keep the speculum in position. It can be used to take smear or for culture and sensitivity of the discharge. Minor operative procedure of cervix can be carried out using this speculum. The difficulty is it obscures inspection of the vaginal walls under direct vision. Of course, while taking out slowly vaginal walls can be inspected.

Before insertion of the speculum the women should be informed about the procedure for her full cooperation. For insertion of the speculum labia are separated with thumb and index finger of the left hand and a well-lubricated speculum is gently introduced inside the vagina. If needed anterior vaginal wall

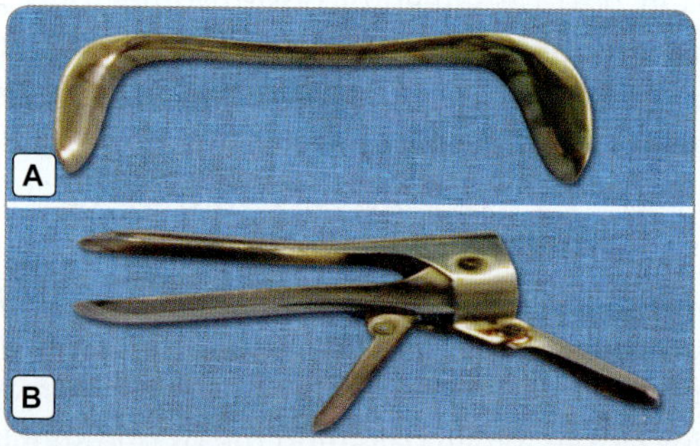

Fig. 10: Common vaginal speculum: (A) Sim's bivalved posterior vaginal speculum; (B) Cusco's speculum

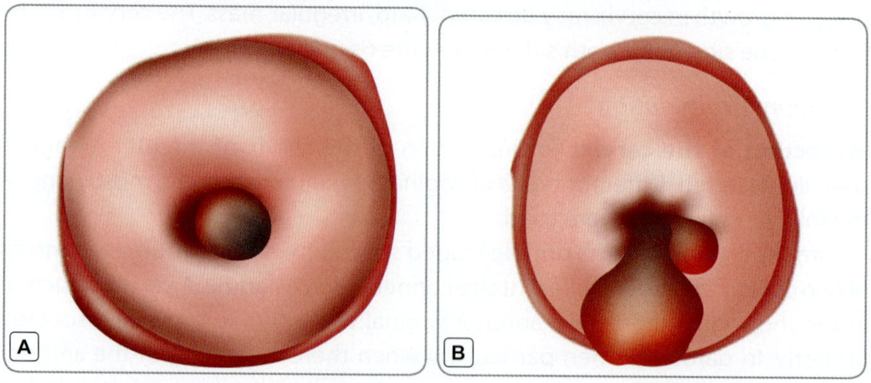

Fig. 11: Cervical polyp

is retracted with the help of the anterior vaginal wall retractor. Then the cervix is inspected for its size, shape, color, smoothness or ulceration, any bleeding on touch or having erosion, presence of prominent vessels, etc, presence of polyp, discharge and bleeding is noted. After inspection of the cervix the vault of vagina is inspected. After examination is over smear from cervix for pap smear or discharge for culture and sensitivity test is taken as indicated and the speculum is gently withdrawn. While withdrawing, the posterior vaginal wall is inspected and the patient is asked to cough or to strain downwards to elicit laxity of the vault or posterior vaginal wall, if any.

Bimanual Examination

Bimanual examination is best performed in dorsal position. It is performed using both hands together. Both index and middle fingers of well-lubricated, gloved right hand are introduced inside vagina. If vagina is narrow examination is performed using the index finger only. Fingers are pushed through the anterior vaginal fornix. The left hand is kept in the anterior abdominal wall in the suprapubic region and gentle counter pressure is applied and organs are palpated between both hands. The purpose of bimanual examination is to determine the size, shape, position and mobility of the uterus. The uterus can be easily felt between both hands when it is anteverted. In retroverted uterus vaginal fingers are pushed through the posterior fornix and the body of the uterus is felt. It should be remembered that when the fingers are pushed through the posterior fornix the patient may feel pain and may resist further examination. If the uterus is enlarged its size and regularity of the surface are noted. Moving the cervix from one side to other its mobility is determined. Next, fingers are pushed through one of the fornices and attempt is made to palpate the adnexa of that side. In normal condition tubes and ovaries are not palpable. Tubes are palpable only following some disease and it may elicit tenderness. If a lump is felt by the side of the uterus its size, shape and consistency are

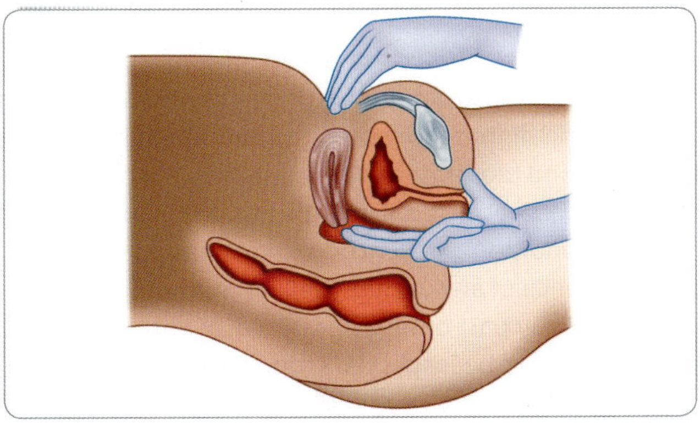

Fig. 12: Bimanual examination

noted. Some lump may be tender on palpation. Mobility of the lump should be noted by fixing the uterus with the vaginal fingers and moving the lump up and down and from side to side by the abdominal hand. When the cervix, i.e. the uterus moves with the movement of the lump, the lump is of uterine origin. A lump not adherent to the uterus does not move with the movement of the cervix. In case of ovarian cyst a definite gap may be felt between the lump and the uterus. A lump may be adherent to the uterus or to the lateral pelvic wall or to the both, thereby restricting its mobility. Again tenderness can be elicited by moving the cervix vaginally form one side to the other.

Sometimes in obese woman it is very difficult to palpate the pelvic organs by bimanual examination. Loaded rectum may give some wrong impression as pelvic tumor. Fecal matter may also create confusion. But fecal matter indents on pressure. After completion of bimanual examination fingers are taken out and the discharge smeared on the fingers should be noted.

Rectal Examination

Rectal examination should be a part of gynecological examination. Lubricated gloved index finger is introduced inside the rectum. First the rectal mucosa is palpated to note the smoothness and mobility. Pushing up in the pelvis a lump, particularly a tumor occupying the pouch of Douglas can be felt easily with the finger in rectum. If present its extent, smoothness of the surface and consistency are determined. Then one should feel for presence of nodular swelling in the pouch of Douglas, which is an important finding in ovarian malignancy. In case of carcinoma of cervix, extension of disease to the parametrium and utero-sacral ligaments can be palpated easily by rectal examination. Sometimes to exactly define the relationship of a swelling to vagina and rectum combined vaginal and rectal examination is carried out. In young virgin girl it is not possible to do vaginal examination without anesthesia. In that case by rectal examination the size, shape, position of the uterus and presence of any abnormal swelling in pelvis can be determined by rectal examination.

Examination of Breast

Examination of breast also should be a part of gynecological examination. During immediate pre-menstrual period there may be mild engorgement of the breasts and may be slight tender on palpation. The patient is asked to sit at the edge of the table and breasts are uncovered, with her hands clasped behind the head and shoulders retracted. First, breasts are inspected for symmetry, contour and skin condition. Presence of skin lesion, erythema, increased vascularity, and presence of any undue swelling is noted. Retracted nipple and dimpling of skin over any part of breast is noted. In case of pendulous breasts the underlying skin should be inspected lifting them with hands.

Palpation

Patient is then asked to keep her hands on her hips and sit comfortably and palpation is carried out methodically. The palmer aspect of the fingers are placed over the center of the breast and moved in an enlarging concentric circles to cover the whole breast. Alternatively the breast is gently squeezed between two hands and the breast is palpated, next an outward traction is applied to palpate the tissues attached to the chest wall. In pendulous breast one hand is kept between the breast and the chest wall and palpation is carried out gently with the other hand. The upper outer quadrant and the axillary tail should be palpated.

Next the lymph nodes should be examined. The woman is asked to raise one hand and the examiner should place his hand in axila, then the women will lower her hand and the examiner will examine the axillary lymph nodes. Then palpation of the supraclavicular gland is performed and the same procedure is repeated on the other side also.

Then the patient is placed in supine position. A pillow is kept under the shoulder to elevate the side to be examined. Arms should be kept over her head. The breast is palpated pressing over the chest wall, with the palmer aspects of the fingers from periphery to center in a clockwise direction. If the patient gives history of discharge from the nipple, attempts should be made to express some discharge for further examination.

The idea of breast examination is to determine tenderness, nodularity and palpable mass in it. In case a mass is detected its size, texture, margin and fixity are determined.

chapter

9 Diagnosis of Pregnancy

Diagnosis of pregnancy depends on certain symptoms and signs. History and clinical examination are supported by laboratory investigations to arrive at a proper diagnosis.

❐ SYMPTOMS OF PREGNANCY

Amenorrhea

Cessation of menstruation is the first symptom of pregnancy. Besides pregnancy amenorrhea may be due to many other causes. These include lactational amenorrhea which may be of short duration, though, sometimes it may be prolonged to 3–6 months. Pregnancy may occur in a lactating mother also. Another cause of secondary amenorrhea is anovulation. In this condition also period of amenorrhea is of short duration. Anxiety and fear of pregnancy also may lead to cessation of menstruation. Regular menstruation does not occur before **menarche** and after menopause, but there are reports of pregnancy occurring during these periods.

Bleeding during very early in pregnancy creates confusion in diagnosis of pregnancy. Some women may have bleeding which she **presumes** to be period of next menstruation, which even may recur almost every month for few months. Sometimes there may be slight bleeding during fusion of the **decidua capsularis** with **decidua vera**. Though this may be a normal phenomenon it is regarded as **threatened** abortion and treated accordingly.

Breast Symptoms

During the first four weeks of pregnancy the woman feels pricking and tightening sensation in breasts due to increased vascularity. In the subsequent weeks breast size enlarges and becomes tense, painful, with sense of fullness. By about 8 weeks of gestation bluish veins are noticeable over the breasts which is more prominent in women of fare complexion. Most of these symptoms are not constant and many women may experience these symptoms during premenstrual period or in case of mastitis.

In the later part of first trimester Montgomery's tubercles become more prominent on the areola. The primary areola enlarges and becomes more dark. **Colostrum** can be expressed by about 16th week of pregnancy and secondary areola appears around the primary one. These breast changes are characteristic in **primigravida** but are less important in **multiparous** women.

Frequency of Micturation

Frequency of **micturation** is a common symptom of early pregnancy. During first trimester the enlarging uterus is still a **pelvic** organ and it presses over the urinary bladder leading to frequency of micturation. Frequency is more common during the day time as the uterus presses over the bladder in standing posture.

Some women complain of incomplete evacuation of bowel. During pregnancy blood concentration of progesterone increases. Progesterone induces relaxation of the smooth muscles of gut resulting in reduced peristalsis and hence incomplete evacuation of bowel.

Tiredness (Malaise)

Tiredness is complained by many during pregnancy. With other symptoms it can be considered for diagnosis of pregnancy.

Abdominal Enlargement

Abdominal swelling becomes evident during the second trimester of pregnancy. Some women, particularly with irregular menstrual cycle, becomes suspicious of pregnancy only when she notices the swelling. Similarly swelling may be there in lower abdomen with ovarian tumor or simply with accumulation of fat.

Sensation of Fetal Movement

Intrauterine fetal activity is appreciated by the women in around 16–20 weeks of pregnancy. The term quickening is used to describe the first fetal movement appreciated by the pregnant women. Many a times a woman confuses bowel movement as movement of the fetus.

Nausea and Vomiting

Nausea and vomiting are very common symptoms of early pregnancy. Nausea appears even before 6 weeks of pregnancy. Sometimes vomiting is excessive and harass the women. These symptoms subside spontaneously by 12 weeks of pregnancy. These are important symptoms of pregnancy but may be present in other causes of gastrointestinal disturbances without pregnancy.

❐ SIGNS OF PREGNANCY

Any of the above symptoms alone is not sufficient to establish the diagnosis of pregnancy. A combination of these symptoms strongly suggest presence of pregnancy. For confirmation positive clinical signs and sometimes laboratory investigations are helpful. Certain clinical signs like palpation of fetal parts, presence of fetal heart sound are confirmatory signs of pregnancy whereas others are only presumptive.

Clinical Signs of Pregnancy

Clinical signs of pregnancy are mostly due to physical changes during pregnancy.

Uterine Sign

Uterine signs are due to changes in the uterus in size, texture and vascularity. Size of the uterus enlarges during pregnancy. In very early weeks of pregnancy uterine enlargement is difficult to ascertain in multiparous women and in women with fatty abdominal wall. Later on when the uterus becomes globular and when there is progressive enlargement diagnosis is more easy.

Another change of the uterus is softening. Softening of the uterus is due to increased vascularity. On bimanual examination a pregnant uterus is felt soft and elastic. The isthmus, the junction between the body of the uterus and the cervix, softens fast which can be elicited by bimanual examination. On the basis of this fact previously Hegar's sign was elicited. To elicit this test one hand is kept in anterior abdominal wall and the fingers of the other hand in vagina. Fingers of both hands are pressed on the soft isthmic part of the cervix. These fingers almost meet because of the softness of the elongated cervix. This sign is no longer practised for fear of inducing miscarriage.

Discoloration of the cervix is another sign which is also due to increased vascularity. Blue discoloration of the cervix and vagina when marked are taken as sign of pregnancy.

Gradual Enlargement of the Uterus

Gradual enlargement of the uterus is an important clue for diagnosis of pregnancy. By about 12 weeks of pregnancy fundus of the uterus is palpable just above the level of the symphysis pubis. With thin abdominal wall the fundus can be felt even at 10 weeks of pregnancy. At 24 weeks the fundus reaches the level above the umbilicus and at 36 weeks reaches the xiphisternum. Afterwards as term pregnancy approaches the fundus drops down to the level of 32 weeks of pregnancy.

Pregnant uterus undergoes spontaneous, painless contraction which can be felt by placing a hand over the uterus. These painless contractions are known as Braxton-Hicks contraction.

Palpation of Fetal Parts

Fetal parts are palpable from about 20 weeks and fetal heart sound is audible by about 24 weeks of pregnancy.

Laboratory Test

Laboratory test for diagnosis of pregnancy depends on presence of beta subunit of human chorionic gonadotropin in urine of pregnant women. Human chorionic gonadotropin is a hormone secreted by the trophoblast tissue of chorionic villi of placenta. Its secretion starts around the time of implantation. Concentration of this hormone can be measured in blood or urine. Urine test for presence of human chorionic gonadotropin (hCG B subunit) is the commonly used method for diagnosis of pregnancy.

The principle of the test is formation of an antigen-antibody complex. Here urinary hCG and an antibody against hCG (Anti-hCG) are used. First this antibody is mixed with urine of the woman to be tested. If she is pregnant her urine contains hCG, which is neutralized by added anti-hCG. Next an indicator, containing hCG coated latex particles or red blood cell is added, which will show no reaction as anti-hCG has already been neutralized. This test is positive.

If the patient is not pregnant there is no hCG in urine to be tested and anti-hCG will be available to react with the indicator. The result is negative.

Nowadays several test kits are available commercially to carry out the test. Monoclonal antibodies against β-hCG have been prepared. These antibodies are tagged with latex particles or red blood cells to carry out agglutination test. These kits show positive reaction with change of color. Urine shows positive reaction with concentration of hCG more than 25 IU/L. Result becomes positive within the first week following missed period.

❐ ULTRASONOGRAPHY

Ultrasonography is rarely used for diagnosis of pregnancy, though diagnosis can be made very early. During ultrasonography the following points are noted.

Identification of the Gestational Sac

Identification of the sestational sac is the earliest sonographic sign of pregnancy. A gestational sac of 2–3 mm corresponding to 4 weeks 1 day to 4 weeks 3 days can be visualized by transvaginal sonography. The gestational sac is surrounded by an echogenic rim of tissue. These echos are due to developing chorionic villi and decidual tissue. Gestational sac size is determined by calculation of the mean sac diameter (MSD). A gestational sac of 5 mm MSD corresponding to 5 weeks of gestational age can be seen at transabdominal sonography. Small sacs are usually round but bigger sac becomes elliptical.

Yolk Sac

The yolk sac is seen as a round-shaped **sonolucent** sac with definite **echogenic** periphery. By transvaginal sonography it is seen as early as 5th week of gestation. Visualization of yolk sac confirms presence of intrauterine pregnancy. By transabdominal route it can be detected by 7 weeks of gestation when **MSD** is 20 mm. The diameter of the yolk sac increases gradually between 5–10 weeks of gestational age to a maximum diameter of 5–6 mm. With advancing gestational age it detaches from the embryo and is not detected sonographically by the end of first trimester.

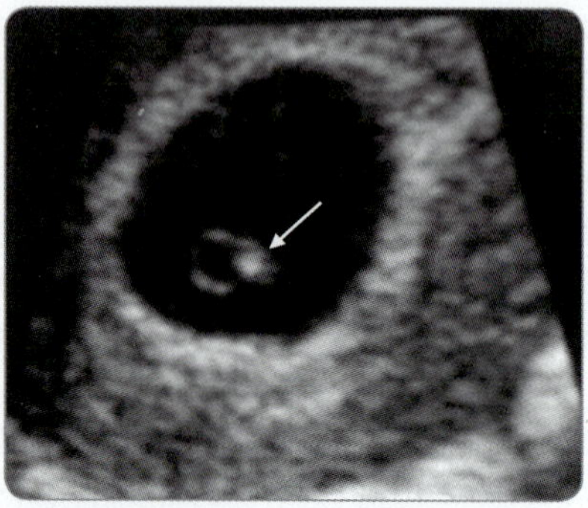

Fig. 1: Ultrasonography showing the early gestational sac with yolk sac

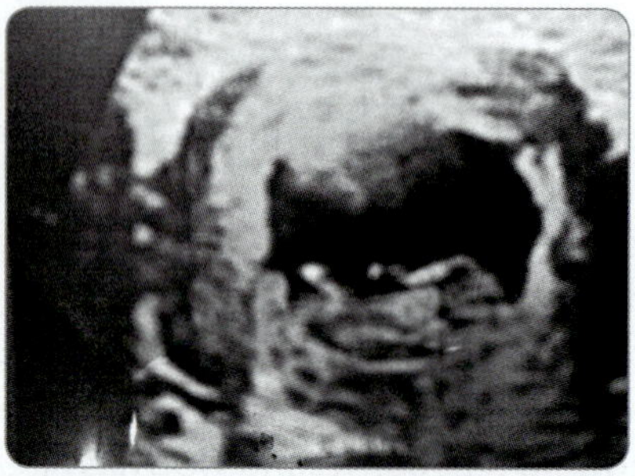

Fig. 2: Ultrasonography of early pregnancy showing fetal limbs

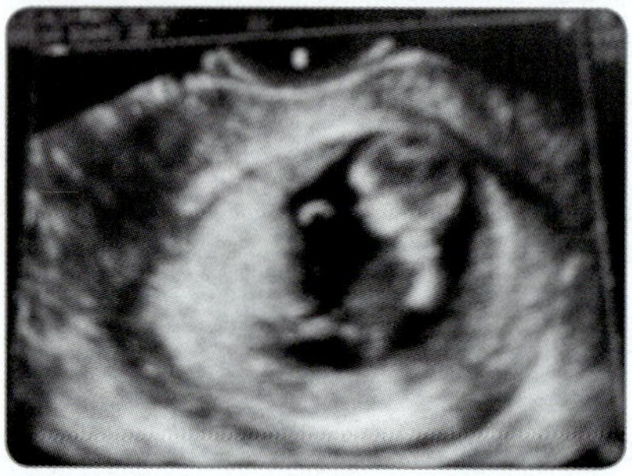

Fig. 3: Ultrasonography of pregnancy – 7 weeks

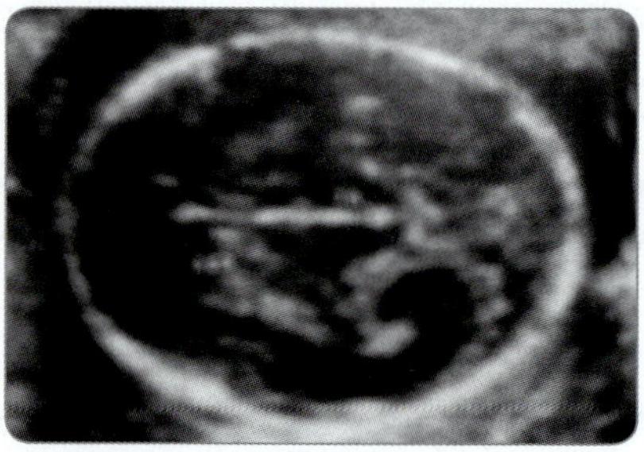

Fig. 4: Fetal skull showing the biparietal diameter

Visualization of the Embryo and Cardiac Activity

Using transvaginal transducer embryo can be detected between 5 and 6 weeks of gestational age. Initially embryonic disc is detected as an area of focal thickening along the periphery of the yolk sac. Cardiac activity is detected at about 6 weeks of gestational age. By trans-abdominal route cardiac activity is detected by 7 weeks of gestation.

During this period of embryonic growth there is dramatic progression of different body parts. The embryo increases in length by about 1 mm per day. By 6 weeks the embryo makes a **ventral** folding. Between 7–8 weeks limb buds appear and by 9 weeks the **extremeties protrude** ventrally. The trunk begins to elongate. By 10 weeks of gestational age the embryo becomes like a human.

Differential Diagnosis

Signs and symptoms of pregnancy, described already, may be present in different other conditions also. Here the condition causing lower abdominal **swelling** will be discussed.

Full Bladder

A full bladder may be confused with pregnant uterus by its position and **cystic** nature. The urinary bladder may be **distended** in the presence of pelvic tumor or by **retroverted gravid** uterus. Catheterization reveals the nature of the swelling. It is always advisable to ask the woman to pass urine before examination.

Uterine Fibromyoma

Uterine fibromyoma causes enlargement of the uterus. A single fibromyoma leads to uniform enlargement of the uterus. As a rule fibromyoma are usually firm in consistency, though it may be soft enough with cystic degeneration to simulate pregnant uterus. The striking feature of fibromyoma is heavy bleeding during menstruation. They are hardly associated with amenorrhea. Urine for pregnancy test is negative in fibromyoma and ultrasonography clearly shows presence of the tumor.

Ovarian Tumor

Ovarian tumor, particularly cystic ovarian tumor occupies the **suprapubic** region in midline. On bimanual examination the uterus of normal size is felt separate from the cyst. Menstrual abnormality is rare with ovarian tumor. Pregnancy test is negative. Ultrasonography of pelvis clearly shows the ovarian tumor with a normal size uterus.

Pseudocyesis (Spurious Pregnancy)

Pseudocyesis or spurious pregnancy is a peculiar but rare condition usually occurs in women desirous of pregnancy or near menopause. It is an imitation of pregnancy. The woman presents all the symptoms and signs of pregnancy. The woman is not amenorrheic but periods are usually irregular. In many women there is morning sickness which may be psychological, some even may present with the enlargement of breast and **galactorrhea.** There may be progressive enlargement of the abdomen. She firmly believes that she is pregnant.

On careful examination the correct diagnosis can be made. On bimanual examination **normal size** uterus is felt. The abdomen becomes flat on administering anesthesia.

❒ SUMMARY OF SYMPTOMS AND SIGNS OF PREGNANCY

8th week: Amenorrhea, morning sickness, bladder irritability, discomfort in breast. Pregnancy test positive.

9th to 12th week: Amenorrhea, morning sickness, bladder irritability, **uterus palpable per abdomen**, softening of cervix, bluish coloration of cervix and vagina, pigmentation of areola.

13th to 20th week: Amenorrhea, quickening, gradual enlargement of uterus, **ballotment,** softening of cervix, pigmentation of areola, **Montgomery's tubercle**, **secondary** areola.

21st to 28th week: Gradual enlargement of the uterus, **fetal heart sound present**, fetal movement felt, **Braxton-Hicks contraction present.**

28th week onwards: Gradual enlargement of uterus with presence of fetal movement and fetal heart sound.

chapter 10

Examination and Observation in Labor

Pregnancy culminates in labor and labor is defined as a process by which the fetus is expelled followed by the placenta. It is difficult to ascertain exactly when labor begins. Duration of labor extends from the onset of painful uterine contraction and lasts during the whole process of expulsion of the fetus and placenta. It is a continuous process till delivery is completed. The major events of labor are gradual dilatation of the cervix, descent of the fetal presenting part and delivery of the baby.

❐ ONSET OF LABOR

The symptoms and signs of onset of labor are – painful uterine contraction, gradual dilatation of cervix and presence of 'show'.

Pregnant uterus exhibits painless, irregular contraction. This irregular contraction can be felt on placing a hand over the uterus. These contractions are not strong enough to elicit pain to be appreciated by the woman. With the onset of labor uterine contractions become painful and regular.

Uterus contracts in a rhythmic manner and the wave of uterine contraction starts in the fundus of the uterus and extends downwards. When it contracts

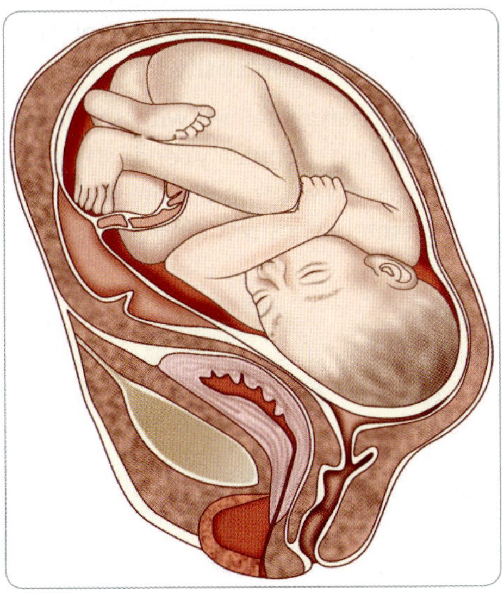

Fig. 1: Term fetus inside the uterus

it contracts as a whole. This is again known as uterine systole. One peculiarity of uterine contraction during labor is that the muscle fibers of myometrium retract or become shorter after each contraction. The upper uterine segment of uterus is more active than the lower uterine segment. As a result of retraction of the muscle fibers of upper uterine segment after each uterine contraction the lower uterine segment and the cervix undergo corresponding dilatation.

During the early stage of labor contractions are weak and infrequent, the interval between two contractions may be 10–20 minutes. Gradually the interval between two contractions reduces and during the second stage of labor it is about 1–3 minutes. Between two uterine contractions the uterus relaxes. It is also known as uterine diastole. In early labor the duration of uterine contraction is short, lasting about 30 seconds, whereas in second stage of labor duration of each contraction increases up to about 90 seconds. Similarly intensity of uterine contraction also increases with advancement in labor being maximum during the second stage of labor.

Pain: Women often report to labor room after onset of labor pain. Pain coincides with uterine contraction of labor and is one of the **three** cardinal signs of labor. The exact time of onset of pain should be asked along with interval between two pains. Duration of uterine contraction and pain is important to notice. Uterine contraction begins before the woman feels pain and gradually intensity of both uterine contraction and that of pain increases, then gradually pain ceases but contraction lasts for some more time. This relation of uterine contraction with pain can be appreciated by placing a hand over the uterus from beginning of a uterine contraction.

Another important feature of uterine contraction and hence of pain is that it is intermittent in nature and the intervening period is pain free. This is essential for the well-being of the mother and the fetus. The woman may experience associated back pain. She usually gives history of shortening of interval between pain along with increase in intensity.

Show: Show is a mucus discharge stained with small amount of blood. The mucus comes from cervix. During pregnancy cervix is filled with a plug of mucus. At the beginning of labor there is widening of the internal os and separation of fetal membranes near the internal os resulting in slight oozing of blood. This

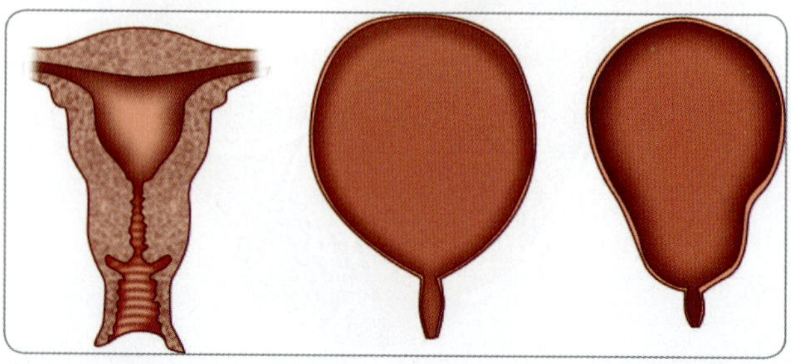

Fig. 2: Increasing size of the uterus with advance of pregnancy

blood is mixed with the plug of cervical mucus and is discharged. 'Show' may precede the onset of labor by several hours or even few days.

❒ DILATATION OF CERVIX

Gradual dilatation of the cervix takes place in labor. It is a sign of labor. At the onset of labor the condition of the cervix is very variable and in few cases it becomes difficult to assess cervical change. As uterine contraction continues cervical changes become evident on vaginal examination. Gradually the cervix starts dilatation.

When the cervix is sufficiently dilated there is no problem for diagnosis of labor.

The term 'ripe cervix' is applied to the cervix which is very soft, partially effaced and slightly dilated. Usually a ripe cervix indicates that labor is going to start.

When the cervix dilates the fetal membranes detach from the adjacent lower uterine segment and with accumulation of **liquor amnii** 'a bag of membrane' is formed. This bag of membrane starts to protrude through the dilated cervical canal. During uterine contraction the bag becomes tense. The bag of membrane is a good cervical dilator.

❒ FALSE LABOR

Before the onset of true labor the woman may experience irregular uterine contraction with discomfort in lower abdomen. False labor is one in which there is irregular painful uterine contraction without cervical change. This type of uterine contraction may continue for some days and ultimately ends in true labor pain or on the other hand pain may subside spontaneously for few days and the woman remains comfortable before true labor starts. False labor pain ceases following an enema or after sedation to the mother.

❒ STAGES OF LABOR

Usually the process of labor is divided into three stages:

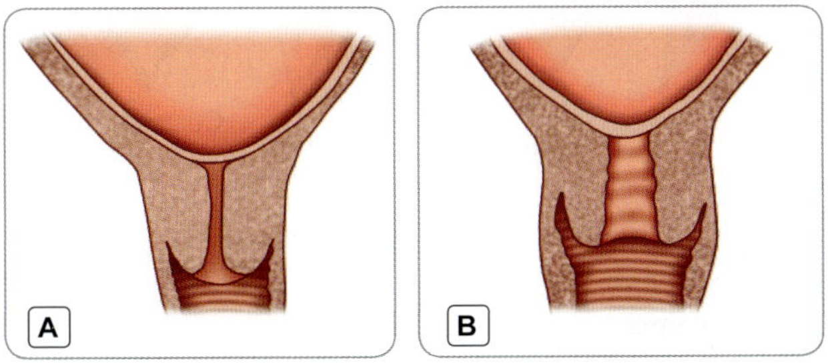

Figs 3A and B: Cervix in pregnancy. (A) Nulliparous; (B) Multiparous

First Stage of Labor

The first stage of labor is from onset of regular, painful uterine contraction to full dilatation of cervix.

At the initial stage uterine contraction is weak and comes at prolonged interval, but gradually it becomes strong and frequent. The main purpose of first stage of labor is dilatation of the lower uterine segment and of the cervix. Contraction and retraction of the longitudinal fibers of uterus slowly dilates the lower uterine segment and opens up the cervix, and the cervix also starts becoming shorter. As the internal os opens the cervix is dilated from above downwards and becomes shorter and shorter. At last no **projection** is felt vaginally and whole of the cervix is taken up with the lower uterine segment. This is known as effacement of cervix. Without complete effacement complete dilatation does not take place. In **multiparous** women the external os often admits one finger before onset of labor. Sometimes the cervix may be shorter and may be completely effaced.

Dilatation of the lower uterine segment and of the cervix causes separation of **amnion** and **chorion** from the adjacent uterine wall. Small amount of liquor **amnii** accumulate there forming a small bag of water or bag of membrane. After further dilatation of the cervix more amount of **liquor ammii** gets accumulated in the bag and during uterine contraction the bag of membrane is forced into the open cervical canal and this helps in further cervical dilatation. At the beginning of an uterine contraction more liquor accumulates in the bag and if the head comes down simultaneously and fits well in the lower uterine segment it separates the liquor in the bag from the liquor amnii remaining

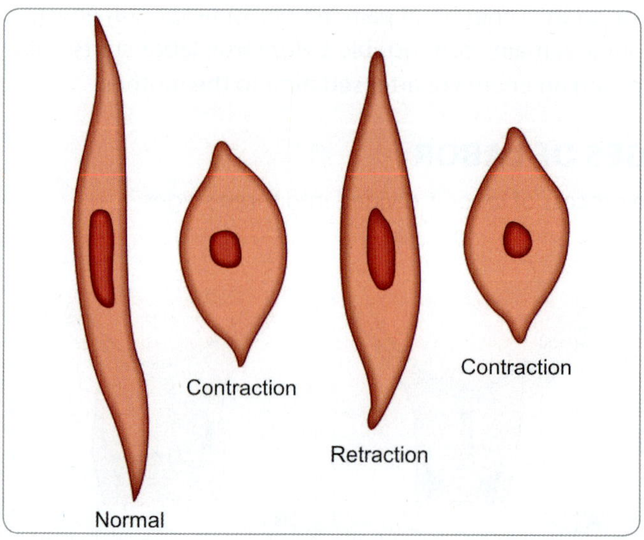

Fig. 4: Changes in uterine muscle fibers during labor

inside the uterine cavity. The liquor amnii in the bag is called forewater and that inside the uterine cavity is hind water.

The first stage of labor is further divided into latent phase and active phase. Latent phase is from the onset of labor upto 3 cm dilatation of the cervix, then the active phase begins. Latent phase is characterized by slow cervical dilatation and of variable duration. During the active phase in primigravida women cervix dilates at the rate of about 1 cm per hour. Along with dilatation of the cervix descent of the presenting part occurs. With strong uterine contraction any deflexion present in the fetal head is corrected and facilitates descent of the head.

❐ GRAPH

First stage of labor ends with full dilatation of the cervix. When dilatation is complete the diameter of the cervical canal is 10 cm. Depending on the rate of cervical dilatation the active phase is further sub-divided into an accelerated phase, a phase of maximum slope and a **decelaration** phase (Fig. 5).

Second Stage of Labor

Second stage of labor begins with full dilatation of the cervix and ends with delivery of the baby. The principal event of second stage of labor is descent of the presenting part through the birth canal till it is delivered. Passage of the presenting part dilates the vagina from above downwards. Before expulsion of the baby the uterus, cervix and vagina becomes a single wide canal. Another noticeable feature of second stage is the initiation of voluntary force of the mother to expel the baby. The onset of each uterine contraction is accompanied by straining or "bearing down" effort of the mother, using the muscles of the anterior abdominal wall and of the diaphragm. Generally, she takes a deep breath, then holding her breath bears down with all her effort. The pains of second stage of labor are frequent, stronger and last longer. Towards the end

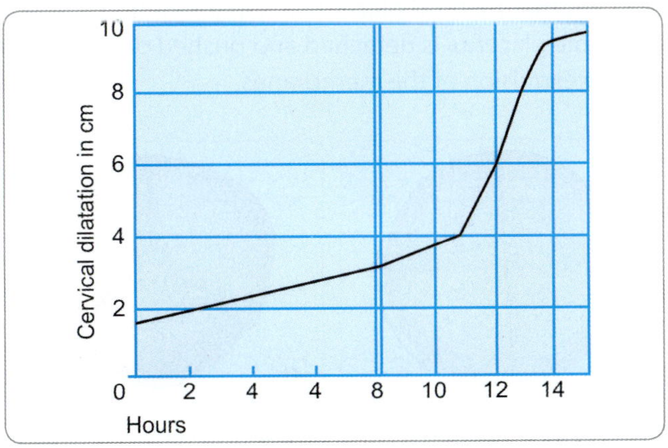

Fig. 5: Cervical dilatation curve

of this stage contraction lasts for about 1–2 minutes and comes at an interval of 2–3 minutes and at the end contractions are almost continuous.

Passing through the birth canal the head presses over the **perineum distending** the vulva. This is called 'crowning' of the head. During the next contraction generally the head is expelled followed by the trunk of the baby.

Rupture of Membranes

The bag of membranes is a good cervical dilator and usually it is ruptured around full dilatation of the cervix. After rupture a gush of clear liquor amnii is discharged. Sometimes, of course, the membranes may rupture during early first stage of labor or very rarely the baby may be born with the membranes intact. Nowadays very often membranes are ruptured artificially to augment labor.

Third Stage of Labor

The third stage of labor is from delivery of the baby to expulsion of the placenta and fetal membranes. After delivery of the baby the uterus becomes smaller in size and the fundus of the uterus reaches upto a level a little below the umbilicus. After expulsion of the baby generally the uterus remains in retracted state without active contraction. During this period if a hand is placed on the uterus a rhythmic painless contraction can be felt. After sometime placenta and membranes are expelled spontaneously.

The uterine walls become thicker and smaller in area along with shrinkage of the placental site, but the placenta remains of the same size and hence detachment must occur. Usually detachment first occurs in the middle of the placenta with a small amount of bleeding which remains between the uterine wall and the placenta.

Following further uterine contraction more placental area is separated followed by bleeding. In this way whole of the placenta is separated and is pulled down the cervical canal. First the placenta is delivered followed by the membranes. In another method placenta is separated from its lower pole and gradually the whole placenta is detached and pushed down the cervical canal to be followed by expulsion of the membranes.

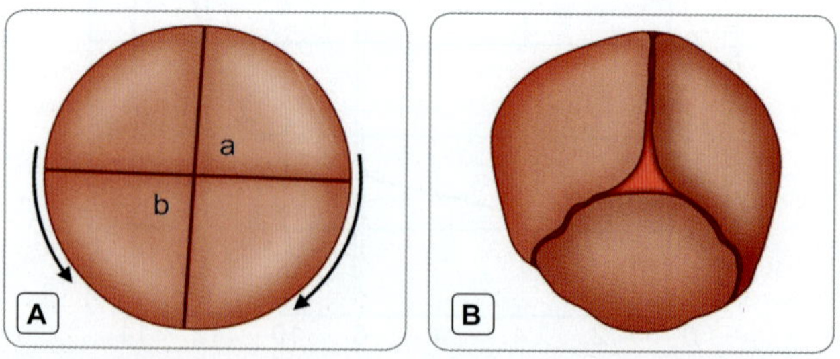

Figs 6A and B: Measurement of fetal skull in vertex presentation. (A) Suboccipitobregmatic diameter – 9.5 cm; (B) Biparietal diameter – 9.5 cm

Expulsion of placenta is followed by a gush of bleeding which is, of course, controlled by adequate contraction of the uterus. If the uterus fails to contract adequately bleeding may follow which needs immediate attention of the physician.

❒ DURATION OF LABOR

Duration of labor may vary considerably from patient to patient. But it is estimated that in a primigravida woman labor lasts on an average 8–16 hours and it is 4–8 hours in a multiparous woman. The average duration of first stage in a primigravida is about 7–11 hours. The duration of second stage in primigravida is around 1 hour and in multiparous woman it is about 20 minutes. The average duration of third stage is about 5–15 minutes.

❒ HISTORY OF TREATMENT RECEIVED OUTSIDE

Usually a patient in labor with or without complication is attended by local doctors. In that case the referral note or the case note sent by the doctor is valuable to know the duration of labor already passed and whether any drug was administered. This valuable piece of document should be attached to the case note of the patient for subsequent review.

❒ EXAMINATION OF THE PATIENT

The procedure for the initial examination of the patient is similar to the examination during antenatal visit. But the initial examination of a patient in labor should be performed by a senior person.

The general condition of the patient is assessed. Pulse is a good indicator of the general condition of the mother in labor. In the initial stage of labor there is no variation in pulse rate. But in a patient with prolonged labor pulse is usually rapid. Patient with bleeding per vaginum may have rapid pulse of low volume. There is a small group of women who show rise of blood pressure for the first time with onset of labor even though she may remain normotensive during pregnancy.

❒ OBSTETRIC EXAMINATION

Abdominal palpation should be performed between two contractions, e.g. during uterine relaxation. Height of the fundus, presentation, position and engagement of the presenting part are assessed carefully. Uterine contraction can be palpated very well by placing the palm of the hand over the abdomen. Detail assessment of uterine contractions is made in respect of frequency, duration and intensity. A careful observation of uterine relaxation is essential as fetal well being during labor depends to a great extent on good uterine relaxation between two contractions. Frequency of uterine contraction is assessed by number of contractions in ten minutes. When three uterine contractions occur during ten minutes labor is said to be established. The duration of contraction is measured in seconds. It is measured from onset of pain in a particular contraction to its cessation. If during the height of a contraction the examining fingers can be dipped over the contracting uterus the intensity is weak and if the uterus becomes hard intensity is strong. During relaxation uterus is not tender.

The size of the fetus and the amount of liquor amnii present is assessed abdominally. Fetal heart sound should be auscultated and counted for two minutes. Initially fetal heart sound should be counted during uterine relaxation. The rate and rhythm should be carefully noted. Then fetal heart rate is checked at the height of contraction and immediately after a contraction. Thereby pathological decceleration of fetal heart is detected. The relation of FHS with uterine contraction is important for further review of the case.

Very often dilatation of intestine is noted during labor particularly in primigravida cases after being in labor for few hours. Dilatation of bowel may increase with progress of labor.

❐ VAGINAL EXAMINATION

Vaginal examination should be minimum to avoid unnecessary bacterial contamination. So, maximum possible information should be obtained from a single examination. The risk of bacterial contamination can be reduced by adopting strict aseptic and antiseptic care. Hands should be washed properly with sufficient soap, drying the hands with sterile towel, sterile hand gloves should be put on. The vulva is swabbed properly with antiseptic solution from above downwards. Then separating the labia with fingers of left hand inner surface of the labia and vestibule are swabbed. A sterile perineal sheet is spread over the abdomen and perineum. Examining fingers are liberally lubricated with antiseptic cream. The index and the middle fingers of the right hand are gently introduced inside the vagina. Utmost care should be taken to avoid undue discomfort to the patient. While making the first vaginal examination following points should be kept in mind and should be sought for systematically so that no valuable point is missed. The following points should be noted:

Cervix: During examination of the cervix, its texture, position in relation to the presenting part, effacement and dilatation are noted.

Presenting part: Determination of the presenting part, in case of cephalic presentation the degree of flexion of the head and thereby the exact presentation and position of the presenting part are noted.

Station of the presenting part is determined in relation to the brim of the pelvis or the ischial spine.

Presence or absence of caput succedaneum is noted.

Presence or absence of fetal membranes is determined. In case membranes are absent color of liquor amnii should be examined.

Next is examination of pelvic architecture .

Condition of vagina and vulva is noted for signs of laceration or infection.

Cervix

During vaginal examination the first thing to examine is the cervix. Cervix during pregnancy is soft in texture but rarely the typical softness of pregnancy may not be felt. The length of the cervix is measured by introducing the index finger inside the cervical canal. The length of an uneffaced cervix is about 2 cm. When cervix is fully effaced the canal is replaced by a mere circular orifice, the margin of which is paper-thin (Fig. 8A). In between these two extremes effacement is expressed in terms of length of the canal compared to the original length.

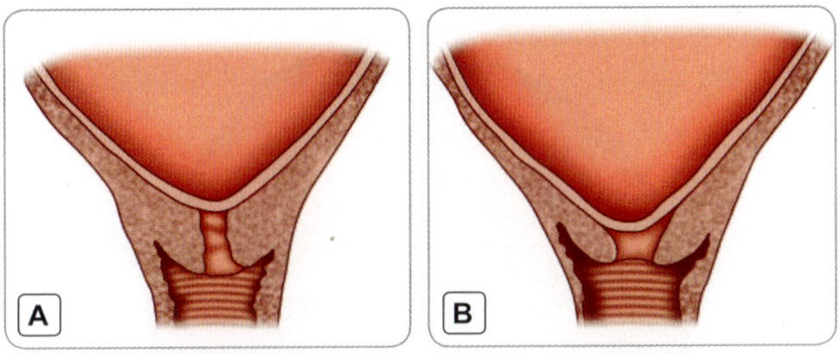

Figs 7A and B: Cervix in early labor: (A) cervix short and internal os dialated; (B) cervix is almost effaced and begins to dialate

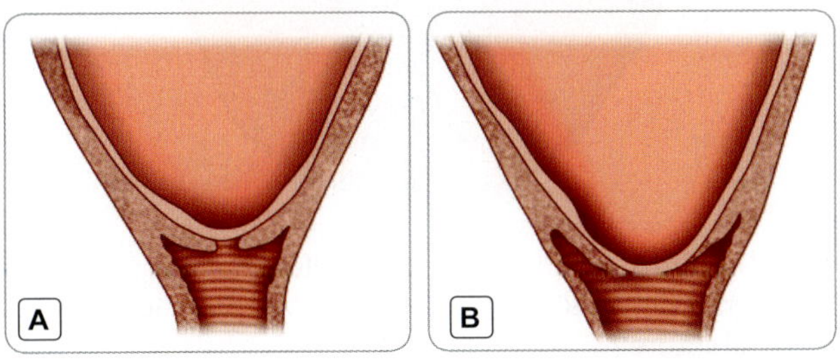

Figs 8A and B: (A) Fully effaced cervix; (B) fully effaced and partially dialated cervix

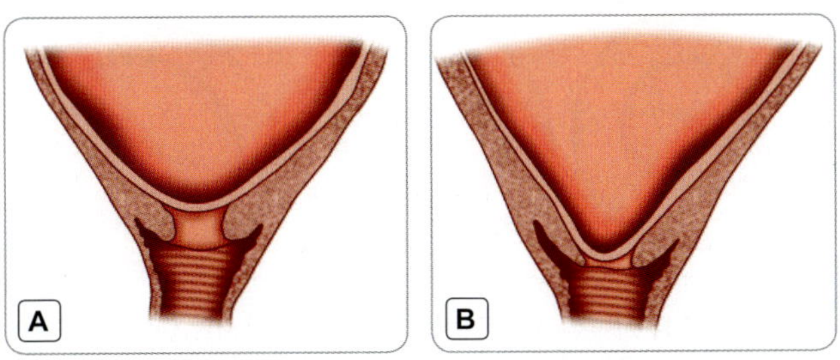

Figs 9A and B: (A) In a multiparous woman cervix ia almost effaced and partially dialated; (B) effaced cervix with partial dialatation

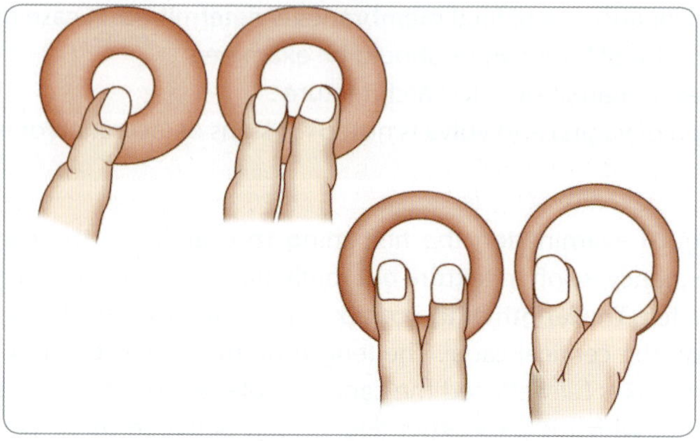

Fig. 10: Assessment of dialatation of cervix (from left) the figures show gradual dialatation and its assessment with the examining fingers

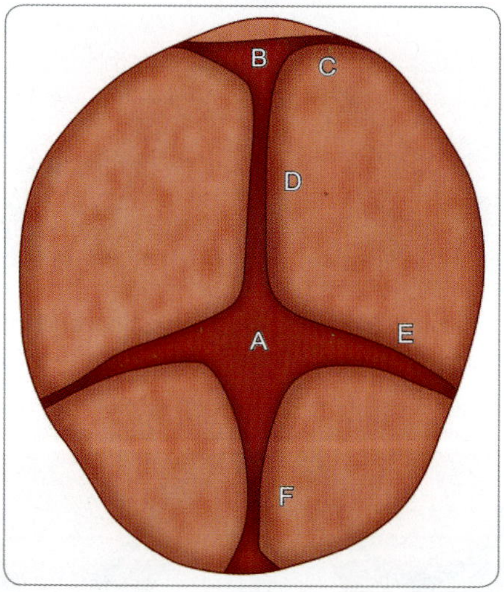

Fig. 11: Fetal skull at term. Note the wide fontanelles and the suture lines: (A) anterior fontanelle, (B) posterior funtanelle, (C) lamboidal suture, (D) sagittal suture, (E) coronal suture and (F) frontal suture

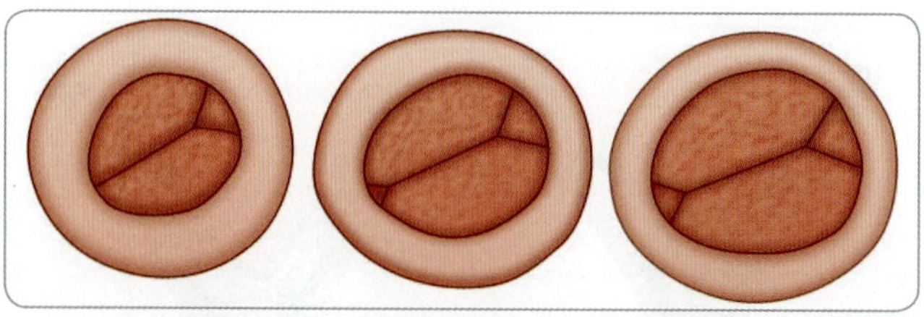

Fig. 12: Assessment of position and flexion attitude of the head in fully-flexed head, the posterior fontanelle is easily felt, when cervix is fully or almost fully dialated, part of the anterior fontanelle may be felt (extreme right)

Cervix dilates gradually as labor progresses. A fully dilated cervix measures 10 cm in diameter. Progressive dilatation of cervix is a good index of progression of labor. In parous women cervix may accommodate 2 fingers (easily) even before the onset of labor, but in primigravida dilatation of the cervix may start at the onset of labor, with or without complete effacement. The examining fingers are stretched transversely so that margins of the fingers touch the edges of the cervix and dilatation is expressed in centimeter.

Position of cervix in relation to the fetal head is important. The cervix may be anterior, posterior or in mid-position.

Mid-position of the cervix is favorable for onset of labor, where as posterior position indicates that the onset of labor will be delayed.

Presenting Part

Next point is to determine the presentation. The different presentations as vertex, face, brow and breech are to be differentiated. The commonest presentation is vertex. In vertex presentation the sagittal suture can be felt lying transversely almost in the midway between the symphysis pubis and the sacral promontory. Vertex presentation and its different positions can be ascertained by the position of suture lines and the fontanelles. It is usually difficult to define the suture lines and the fontanelle if the cervix is not sufficiently dilated and membranes are intact. After examination of the cervix is over, fingers are gently pushed in to touch the presenting part. Fingers are swept from anterior to posterior aspect and in vertex presentation the sagittal suture can be located. Then the sagittal suture is followed on either side. On one side it ends in the posterior fontanelle and on the other is the anterior fontanelle. The anterior fontanelle can be recognized by its lozenge shape, soft membranous floor which is slightly depressed from the surface of the scalp and four sutures running from its angles. The posterior fontanelle is a triangular depressed area and is connected with three sutures. In a premature fetus an unossified membrane may be felt at the posterior fontanelle. The three sutures, the sagittal suture and two lambdoidal sutures should be carefully identified by following the suture lines from the fontanelle. In a fully flexed head the posterior fontanelle is felt easily and it is difficult to feel the anterior one. But in a deflexed head the anterior fontanelle also can be felt. Care should be taken so that the posterior angle of the anterior fontanelle is not mistaken with the posterior fontanelle. The position of the posterior fontanelle in relation to the different quadrant of the pelvis should be determined (Figs 13A–C).

Station

It is important to identify the level of the presenting fetal part inside the birth canal. In an unmoulded head if the lowermost part of the presenting part is at the level of the ischial spine, head is said to be at zero station and the head is engaged. The pelvis is divided into two halves, above and below the level of

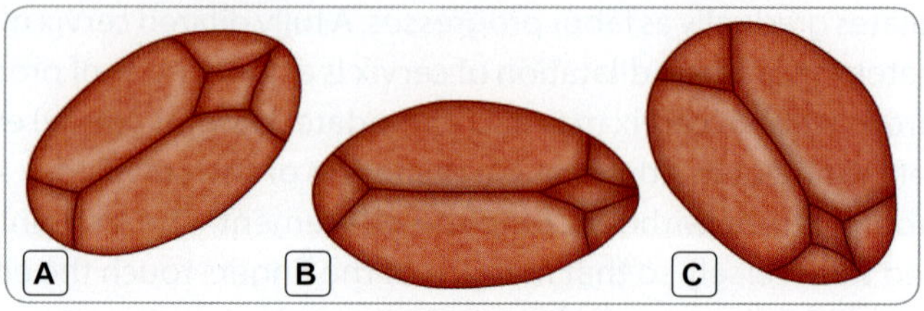

Figs 13A to C: Different position of occiput. (A) right occipito anterior; (B) right occipito lateral and (C) right occipito posterior

the ischial spine. Both halves are divided into five levels. Distance between two of these levels is about 1 cm.

If the presenting part is at the level of the pelvic brim, it is –5 station, if it has descended to a level about 1 cm above the ischial spine (0 station) it is at –1 station. When the presenting part is at the level of the ischial spine it is at 0 station. Similarly if the presenting part is 2 cm below the level of the ischial spine, it is at +2 station, in this manner +3, +4 and +5 station. When the presenting part reaches the perineum, it is at +5 station.

Presence or Absence of Membranes

The tense bulging bag of membranes can be felt during uterine contraction. If uterus is not contracting or between contractions the membranes remain in contact with the presenting part. Rupture of membranes can be diagnosed if the hairs of scalp can be recognized. Diagnosis of ruptured membranes is easy if the examiner can feel or see liquor coming out through the cervix. But it should be remembered that sometimes even with intact membranes liquor may be seen escaping. This may happen with high rupture of membranes.

Color of Liquor Amnii

If membranes are ruptured color of the liquor amnii should be noted. Normally liquor amnii is colorless, though some white flakes may be there. Meconium passed by the fetus mixes with the liquor and change the color to brownish green. Meconium staining of liquor is regarded as a sign of fetal distress.

Caput Succedaneum

Caput succedaneum is one of the changes that takes place in the fetal head during labor. The lower most portion of the head is free from pressure, whereas the surrounding part is pressed upon by the maternal soft tissue like the cervix before its full dilatation and then the pelvic floor.

The pressure interferes with the venous return resulting in effusion of the serous fluid into the subcutaneous space of the pressure-free area of the head. Collection of effusion forms a swelling and it is known as caput succedaneum. Caput is usually formed after rupture of membranes. Presence of a big caput is a sign of prolonged first stage of labor. It is felt as a soft swelling through which it is difficult to palpate the cranial bones and the suture lines.

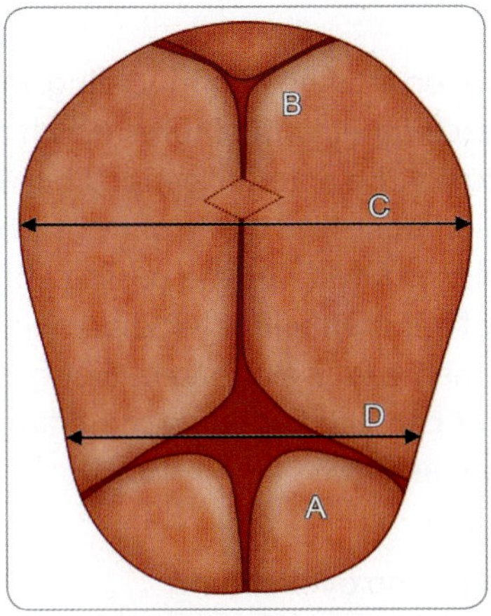

Fig. 14: Fetal skull showing position of (A) anterior fontanelle, (B) posterior fontanelle, (C) bi-parietal diameter, (D) bi-temporal diameter

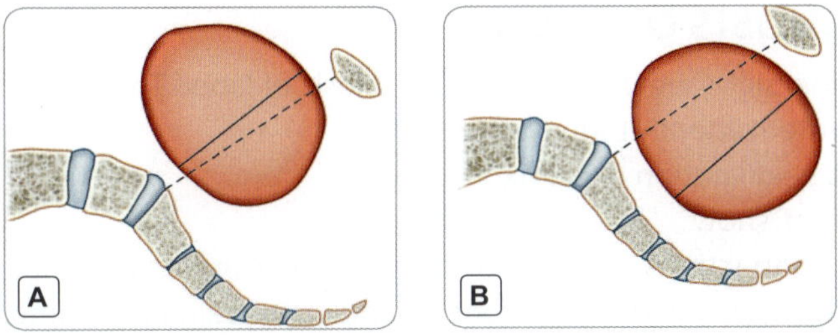

Figs 15A and B: (A) Bi-parietal diameter of the fetal head is above the plane of the pelvic brim-head is not engaged; (B) Bi-parietal diameter of the fetal head is below the plane of the pelvic brim-head is engaged

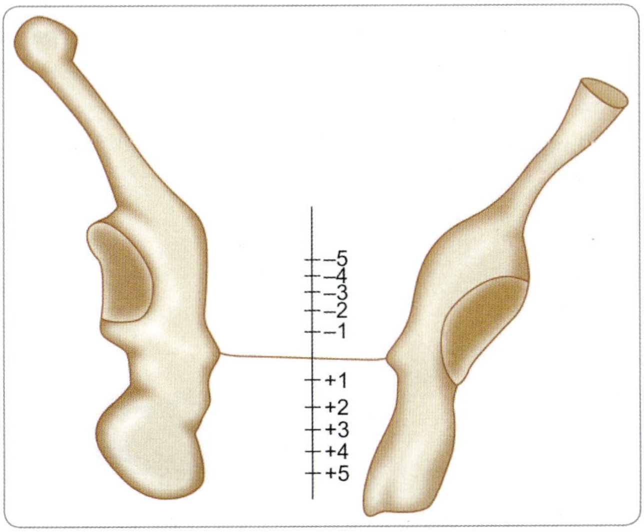

Fig. 16: Station of the fetal head (in fifth). The transverse line indicates the level of the ischial spine (0 – station)

Moulding

Another effect of pressure on fetal head is moulding. In fetal head the bones of the vault are joined to each other with sutures which allows some movement between each other. Usually the anterior parietal bone overlaps the posterior and margin of the occipital bone and rarely of frontal bones are pushed under the parietal bones. Moulding facilitates the passage of the fetal head through the bony pelvis in cases of mild cephalopelvic disproportion. After considerable moulding the shape of the head is elongated. Elongation occurs in the plane right angle to the girth of contact. Excessive moulding may cause intracranial injury. Moulding is graded as:

– Bones normally separated.
+ Suture lines are closed but no overlapping
+ + Overlapping of suture lines but reducible
+ + + Overlapping of suture lines and irreducible.

❒ DIAGNOSIS OF LABOR

Three cardinal signs are described for diagnosis of labor. These are:
- Painful, intermittent uterine contraction
- Progressive dilatation of cervix
- Presence of 'show'.

Uterine contractions in labor come at regular interval and duration and intensity, gradually increases. Patient complains of pain in abdomen and back during each uterine contraction. Along with uterine contractions if the cervix shows sufficient dilatation the diagnosis of labor is confirmed. Presence of show even without sufficient cervical dilatation confirms labor. With passage of time cervix shows progressive dilatation. Sometimes it may not be possible to ascertain onset of labor during the initial evaluation of the patient. In such

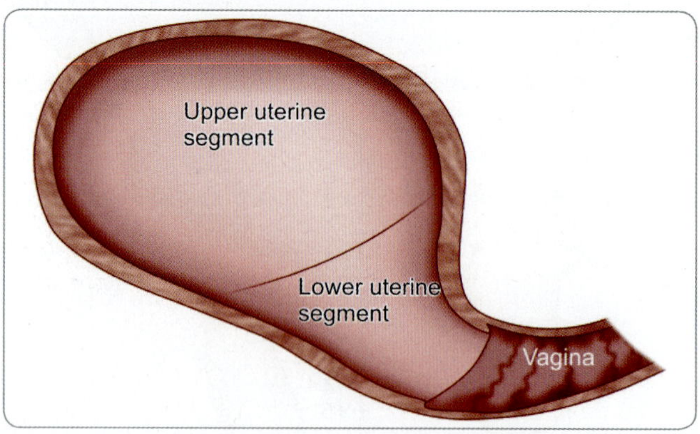

Fig. 17: The birth canal during labor. Uterus, cervix and vagina are converted into a single canal

situation the patient is kept under observation and re-evaluation is done after about 6 hours. In this condition, the fact should be explained to the patient to build her confidence and morale.

Sometimes a patient may come only with draining of clear fluid per vaginum without painful uterine contraction or dilatation of cervix. Then also the patient should be dealt with as in labor.

Observation in Labor

Labor is a physiological phenomenon. In maximum number of cases it follows its normal course and the baby is delivered without much difficulty. But in some cases there may be difficulty. The baby may be depressed with low Apgar score at birth. Sometimes even the mother may be at danger. One can avoid these untoward events provided a constant supervision is maintained by a skilled personnel. Moreover during labor a woman needs adequate psychological support. To build up her morale a doctor or midwife should always be near her and whenever possible the husband or a near relative should be allowed to stay with her in the first stage observation room.

The aims of supervision during labor are to assess (a) the progress of labor, (b) the maternal condition and (c) the fetal condition. It s not possible to lay any time bound schedule how often a parturient mother should be examined. In otherwise normal cases it is a general rule to assess the maternal condition every 1–2 hours and fetal condition is assessed every 15 minutes during the first stage of labor.

Assessment of Maternal Condition

Depending on the condition, the mother is examined hourly or 2 hourly. Pulse, blood pressure, degree of hydration are assessed. In hypertensive woman blood pressure should be recorded every hour or more frequently. Blood pressure should be recorded in between two uterine contractions. If temperature is found to be high during initial evaluation it should be repeated 4 hourly. Recording of temperature is essential for those who come with ruptured membranes.

A patient in labor is administered sedation, intravenous fluid and sometimes antibiotics. Careful note of all these medications, nature of intravenous fluid and amount infused should be kept. Amount of urinary output is also noted. Urine should be tested for proteinuria, particularly in hypertensive women, and for ketone bodies when labor is likely to be prolonged or if the patient is dehydrated.

Assessment of Fetal Condition

Fetal heart should be checked every 15 minutes during the first stage of labor and every 5 minutes during the second stage of labor. Fetal heart sound should be counted before, at the height of, and immediately after uterine contraction. Change in the rate of fetal heart sound immediately after uterine contraction is ominous for fetal health. When deceleration of fetal heart rate immediately after uterine contraction is persistent fetal distress is likely to occur. If fetal tachycardia is detected maternal pulse rate should be counted simultaneously to avoid confusion. In doubtful cases it is better to monitor fetal heart electronically along with fetal blood gas analysis wherever possible.

Assessment of Progress of Labor

Progress of labor is assessed by progressive dilation of the cervix and descent of the fetal presenting part.

The main event of first stage of labor is dilatation of the cervix. Cervical dilatation is described in two phases – latent phase and active phase. Latent phase is upto 3 cm dilatation. This much dilatation is attained within 8 hours of initiation of uterine contraction. If it is prolonged beyond 8 hours it is abnormal and termed as delayed latent phase. After latent phase is over active phase begins. In a primigravida woman the rate of dilatation of the cervix in active phase is about 1 cm per hour. In a multiparous woman dilatation is more quick.

Descent of the presenting part can be assessed abdominally, but to know the exact level vaginal examination is needed. On vaginal examination care should be taken to assess the level of the presenting part in relation to the level of the ischial spine. Besides determining the level, attempt should be made to detect the position of the presenting part.

Uterine Contraction

Good uterine contraction is a pre-requisite of satisfactory progress of labor. While assessing uterine contraction the examiner should evaluate the frequency, duration and intensity of contraction. Frequency is better expressed as the number of contractions in 10 minutes period. Keeping the palm of the hand on the uterus the duration of contraction is assessed. And when the contraction is strong the examining fingers cannot indent the uterus.

Vaginal Examination During Labor

As has been seen vaginal examination is needed to assess progress of labor. But how often it should be done? It should always be remembered that during labor vaginal examination should be minimum to prevent introduction of infection and to ensure comfort to the patient. But it should be performed whenever indicated. A vaginal examination should be performed following rupture of membranes to exclude cord prolapse particularly when the presenting part is not engaged. Again the examination should be repeated at the onset of second stage of labor.

The second stage of labor is from full dilatation of the cervix to delivery of the child. Onset of second stage of labor can be guessed from the beginning of bearing down effort of the woman. In second stage uterine contraction is more frequent and more forceful. The average duration of second stage in primigravida is one hour and in multiparous woman it is about half an hour.

Duration of Labor

It is not easy to calculate the duration of different stages of labor, particularly those of first and second stage in a particular case. The exact time of onset of labor is difficult to know, similarly is the onset of second stage and hence the duration of labor. On an average the duration of first stage in a primigravida is about 10 hours and in a multigravida it is about 5 hours. The second stage in the former is about 1 hour and in the latter it is about 30 minutes and the third stage is about 5–15 minutes in both.

❐ PARTOGRAM

Partogram is a graphic representation of different events of labor. This is a composite labor record where all the details of the progress of labor, maternal condition, fetal condition and drug used are plotted in a single piece of paper against the time scale. From this graph the obstetrician can have an idea of the case at a glance.

Components of labor Graph

In partograph the following points are noted:

Identification of the Patient

Name, age, hospital no., parity, expected date of delivery and date of admission are noted on the top of the partogram. Time of rupture of membrane is also noted on the right hand corner of the top.

Time

The time of admission into labor room is taken as zero hour.
Recordings from above downwards are as follows:

Fetal heart rate recording: Fetal heart rate is recorded on initial examination (zero hour) and at an interval of 30 minutes. The baseline heart rate is plotted. The normal range of fetal heart rate is taken as 120–160 beats per minute. Heart rate above 160 is taken as tachycardia and below 120 beats per minute is taken as bradycardia. The rhythm of the heart beat is noted as regular or irregular accordingly. Fetal heart rate should be recorded in relation to uterine contraction. When deceleration occurs an arrow is drawn to the level of the descent of decceleration and recorded `E' (early), if the rate returns to baseline before the end of the contraction and recorded `L' (late) if there is delay in return.

Liquor: In the column liquor, observation is recorded as `i' if the membranes are intact. If the membranes are ruptured and the draining liquor is clear, it is `C' and `M' if the liquor is meconium stained. Blood stained liquor is marked as `B'. The time of rupture of membranes is noted and also whether done artificially or occurred spontaneously. If the membranes are ruptured on admission, the duration is noted at the beginning.

Moulding: Moulding of the head is recorded as 0, +, ++ and +++.

It is an important sign of cephalopelvic disproportion.

Caput: Caput succedaneum is represented by +, ++, +++ depending upon the size of the caput.

In the middle portion of the graph progress of labor is recorded under the headings of cervical dilatation and descent of the head. Cervical dilatation is drawn from 0–10 cm.

The left part of the graph is for latent phase of 8 hours or till 3 cm dilatation of the cervix. The right half is for active phase and the second stage of labor.

Alert line: In the active phase portion of the graph, a line is drawn from 3 cm dilatation, upwards at a slope of 1 cm per hour to full dilatation. This is alert line. This line alerts the obstetrician of delayed progress.

Action line: This is another line drawn 2 hours to the right of the alert line. This line indicates need for intervention and it is termed action line.

When a patient is admitted with less than 3 cm dilatation of cervix that is in latent phase of labor `X' mark is put at the extreme left of the graph. This is zero time. The curve is then taken forward after 4 hourly vaginal examination. When 3 cm dilatation is achieved the curve is brought to active phase with a curved line to the appropriate place on the alert line. Subsequent recordings are plotted from this point. If a patient is admitted in active phase recording starts on the alert line corresponding to the cervical dilatation and that point is regarded as zero time. In active phase progress should be parallel to the alert line. If the rate of cervical dilatation crosses the alert line the case should be reviewed by a senior obstetrician. If needed labor is accelerated with artificial rupture of membranes or oxytocin drip or both.

Uterine contraction during latent phase is not well established and it may be prolonged without much adverse effect on the mother and the fetus. For this reason nowadays latent phase is omitted in the modern labor graph (Fig. 18).

Descent of the Head

Descent of the fetal head is noted as a descending line in the graph from 5 cm to 0 cm. The station of the head is ascertained half hourly. Then station of the head is best measured by abdominal palpation as the number of fifths the head is above the pelvic brim. When the head is entirely above the brim it is five-fifths above and head that is four-fifths above is just entering the brim. When the head is three-fifths above the brim the examining hands can still go round the head. When more than half of the head enters the brim the hands

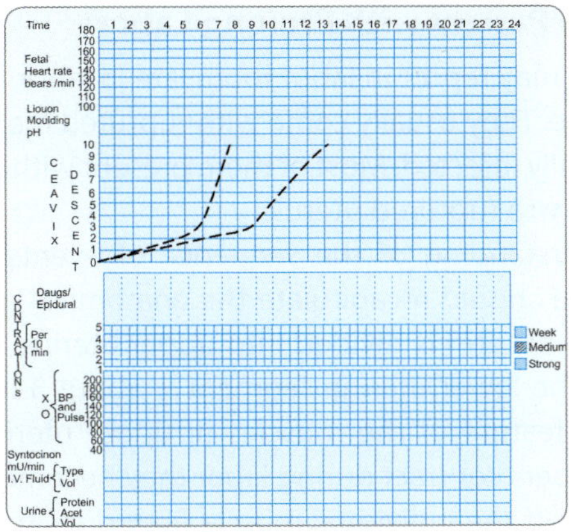

Fig. 18: The partogram

splay outwards. In one-fifth above, only the sinciput can be felt and when no bony points can be felt the head is entirely inside the pelvis. The number of fifths is plotted as `0' on the graph.

Uterine Contraction

Uterine contraction is observed during the last ten minutes of every half hour period. Number of contractions per 10 minutes are represented by the number of blocks on the graph. Duration of contraction is measured in seconds. When the contraction lasts for less than 20 seconds the blocks are filled with dots, cross hatched if duration is less than 40 seconds and blacked out if more than 40 seconds.

Drugs and Intravenous Fluids

These are recorded in the space provided in the graph.

Oxytocin Stimulation

When oxytocin is used to stimulate uterine contractions this can be recorded in the two lines provided indicating the dose and rate of infusion.

Maternal Condition

Maternal conditions like pulse, blood pressure, temperature are recorded in the lower part of the graph.

Urine

The volume of urine and presence or absence of albumin and acetone are recorded every time urine is passed.

Partograph recordings are continued in second stage of labor till delivery of the child and recorded in the graph

Examination of a Patient with Prolong Labor

Sometimes patient may report in labor room late in labor after being in active labor for a long time. They usually come with ruptured membranes and hence infected or potentially infected. Most of them present with signs of obstruction or even may come with ruptured uterus.

For better understanding of the sequence of events that take place in prolonged labor we should recapitulate the anatomical aspect of the uterus at term. The uterus at term is divided into upper uterine segment and lower uterine segment. The lower uterine segment is about 3 inches long at term. One characteristic feature of the muscles of upper uterine segment is that when the muscle fibers contract during labor they become short, but after the contraction passes off the individual muscle fiber does not regain its original length. There remains some amount of shortening of the muscles fibers. So after each successive contraction the muscle fibers become shorter and thicker. This phenomenon is called retraction. Thickening of the upper uterine segment is accompanied by thinning and dilatation of the lower uterine segment. So that the upper uterine segment tries to expel the baby and the lower uterine segment receives the baby before its expulsion through the lower genital tract. As a result the upper and lower uterine segments become distinct from one another, but it cannot be detected by abdominal examination.

When there is insuperable obstruction to the passage of the baby through the lower genital tract obstructed labor results. In this situation the upper uterine segment will go on contracting and retracting in an effort to expel the baby and the lower uterine segment will go on thinning and dilating. At this stage the junction between the upper and lower uterine segments becomes visible as a ring, through the anterior abdominal wall. It can be palpated as a groove running transversely. Formation of the ring is the result of exaggeration of the physiological process of labor. The ring is known as Bandl's ring or retraction ring. If the process continues the upper segment becomes more thick and the lower segment becomes more and more thin and dilated, the ring appears to rise higher and higher. If the obstruction is not relieved lower segment will go on dilating and at one time it ruptures. The rent starts at the lower segment and extends into the upper segment, even upto the fundus. In some cases the rent extends down wards involving upto vagina.

In some cases particularly in primigravida cases the exhausted uterus goes into secondary inertia. In these cases uterine contraction ceases completely. After the period of inertia is over strong uterine contraction starts again.

❒ CLINICAL EXAMINATION

For simplicity of description the patients can be divided into three groups as:

a. Prolonged labor without signs of obstruction.
b. Prolonged labor with signs of obstruction or obstructed labor.
c. Ruptured uterus.

Prolonged Labor Without Signs of Obstruction

In the first group the patient gives history of labor for a considerably long time. There is usually early rupture of membrane. On examination there is tachycardia, dehydration and may be associated with slight rise of temperature. On abdominal examination uterine contraction of variable intensity is present. Normal characteristic of uterine contraction is maintained. Abdomen is not tender. As a result of early rupture of membranes most of the liquor amnii are drained out and the uterus seems to be moulded upon the fetus. The presenting part may or may not be engaged. There may be abnormal presentation or occipito posterior position of vertex presentation. Fetal heart sound is usually present. On vaginal examination vagina is hot and dry. Cervical dilatation may not be complete. An incompletely dilated cervix may not be in contact with the presenting part. The cervix may be found to be hanging like a curtain. Due to early rupture or membranes there is a big caput succedaneum. Moulding may or may not be there.

The above mentioned clinical picture is seen in early cases of obstructed labor also. So when the patient is first examined every attempt should be made to exclude cephalo-pelvic disproportion. Other causes giving rise to this condition are abnormal presentation and occipito-posterior position of vertex presentation.

Prolonged Labor with Signs of Obstruction (Obstructed Labor)

In this condition the patient is anxious with rapid pulse, dry tongue and slight rise of temperature. Urine is usually of high color and shows ketone bodies. Rhythmic strong uterine contraction is there. Uterine contraction maintains its normal rhythmic nature. Contractions come frequently and intensity is strong. The upper uterine segment is retracted and the lower uterine segment is dilated. The Bandl's ring can be felt easily and with passage of time it moves upwards.

Presenting part is usually not engaged and fetal heart sound may be absent. On vaginal examination vagina is hot and dry, cervix is fully dilated. Head is not engaged. There are big caput succedaneum and excessive moulding of the head. The moulded head gets jammed into the pelvis and becomes conical. Due to moulding and caput succedaneum scalp may be visible just above the introitus though major part of the head remains above the brim.

Ruptured Uterus

Rupture of the uterus is a grave condition with high maternal mortality. Rupture usually occurs as a sequele of obstructed labor. But, less frequently rupture may occur even during pregnancy. Rupture is said to be complete when uterine musculature and the peritoneal coat are involved and incomplete when peritoneal layer is intact.

Rupture of the Uterus During Pregnancy

Rupture of the uterus during pregnancy is very rare. Spontaneous rupture of the uterus occurs late in pregnancy and may be due to rupture of previous caesarean section scar and very rarely it may follow a myomectomy operation or a scar following injury during previous curettage. Before actual rupture of the previous caesarean section scar occurs the patient complains of pain over the suprapubic region. It is a good practice to palpate the suprapubic region in cases of post caesarean pregnancy, particularly in late pregnancy, to elicit tenderness. Definite tenderness over a particular area is a danger sign.

Rupture of Uterus During Labor

Obstructed labor is the commonest cause of rupture of the uterus during labor followed by rupture of previous caesarean section scar. Severity of the condition and hence the presenting symptoms and signs depend upon the amount of internal hemorrhage.

Patient usually gives history of protracted labor with strong pains followed by a sensation of "something giving away". This is followed by acute pain in lower abdomen and fainting attack. On initial recovery she may feel cessation of pain. When internal hemorrhage is severe the patient goes into shock. On the other hand in incomplete rupture or rupture of previous caesarean section scar constitutional symptoms may be less severe.

On examination the patient is anxious with rapid pulse of low volume and low blood pressure. Pallor is usually marked. On abdominal examination abdomen is uniformly enlarged without definite contour of the uterus of term size. Bowel is distended, there is evidence of fluid (blood) in peritoneal cavity. Fetal parts are easily palpable. The retracted uterus is felt on one side. On vaginal examination cervix is found to be reformed, presenting part is not accessible and there is blood in vagina. For confirmation of the diagnosis rarely examination under anesthesia is necessary.

chapter

11 Pelvic Assessment

The true pelvis is bounded anteriorly by the pubic bones, laterally by the iliums and posteriorly by the sacrum. Different planes of the pelvis are described which the fetal head is to cross during the process of delivery. Various diameters of these planes are important. Variation of these diameters influences the shape of the pelvis. But in clinical practice, available space inside the pelvis is more important than the actual size and shape. The fetal head is the best pelvimeter. When the head is engaged it is sure that there is no disproportion at the brim.

Clinical assessment of the pelvis is done after 37 weeks of gestation, because by this time the pelvic joints and ligaments attain maximum mobility.

Patient should be in dorsal position. Vulva and perineum are swabbed and wrapped with sterile linen. Well-lubricated index and middle fingers of the examiner are introduced inside the vagina and assessment is done in a systematic way. At first the coccyx is palpated and its mobility is determined. Then the fingers are pushed upwards along the anterior surface of the sacrum. The sacrum is palpated from below upwards and from side to side. Normally the sacrum is slightly concave anteriority. In abnormal state the sacrum may be straight or there may be undue prominence on the anterior surface. Usually the sacrum can be felt upto the 3rd vertebra only.

Next an attempt is made to feel the sacral promontory. In a pelvis of average size the promontory cannot be reached. When the promontory is reached the tip of the middle finger should be kept there and the base of the fingers are pressed against the lower border of the symphysis pubis, and with the index finger of the left hand the point is marked. Then taking out the fingers the distance from the tip of the middle finger to the mark is measured. This gives the diagonal conjugate of the brim. By subtracting 1.5 cm from the diagonal conjugate, the true conjugate can be found out. This is the only diameter of the pelvic brim which can be clinically measured.

After attempting the sacral promontory, fingers are swept laterally to have an idea about the lateral pelvic walls. In a gynecoid pelvis the side walls are almost straight whereas in an android type of pelvis these are almost convergent. The classical description of the gynecoid pelvis is a short section of a 'long cone' and android pelvis is a long section of a 'short cone'. Next is to assess the width of the sacrosciatic notch, which is done by placing the examining fingers over the sacrospinous ligament. Normally two fingers are easily accommodated there.

If this ligament is short it can be assumed that the sacrum is more forward reducing the capacity of the hind pelvis.

Clinically, it is not possible to measure the interspinous diameter which forms the transverse diameter of the least pelvic plane. If the spines are not prominent, side walls are not convergent and spines are placed well apart, it can be assumed that this important diameter is adequate. Of course, with experience one can easily make an idea.

The anteroposterior diameter of the outlet is measured from lower border of symphysis pubis to the tip of the sacrum or the tip of the coccyx, if the later is

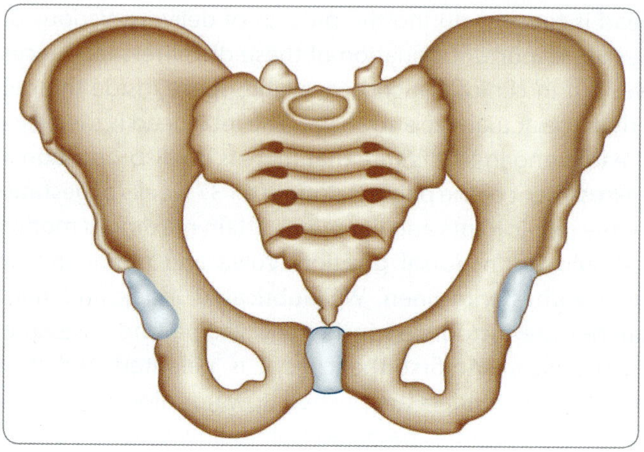

Fig. 1: Female pelvis (anteroposterior view). Note the round shape of the brim and wide sub-pubic angle

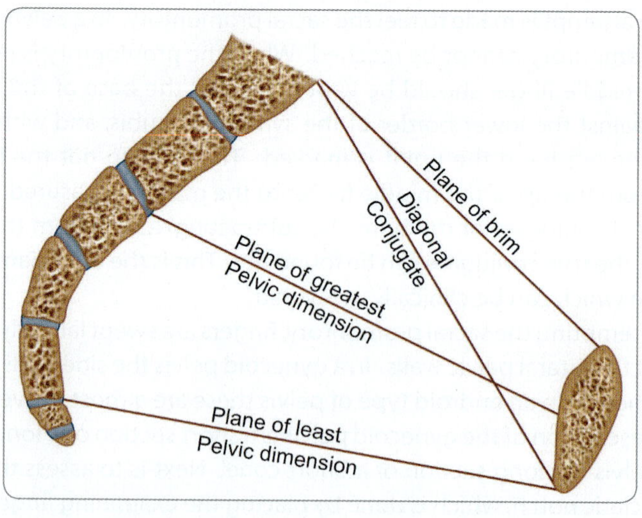

Fig. 2: Different planes of the bony pelvis

fixed. Before taking out the fingers the subpubic angle is assessed by putting the palmer aspect of the fingers at the pubic arch. Normally it is wide and measures more than 90 degree, which easily accommodates the fingers. The transverse diameter of the outlet, i.e. the intertuberous diameter is measured by putting the knuckles between the medial aspects of the tuberosities in front of the rectum. Normally it accommodates four knuckles.

The whole procedure gives a fair idea of the size and shape of the pelvis and with an average size baby vaginal delivery can be expected. But in doubtful cases X-ray pelvimetry may be needed.

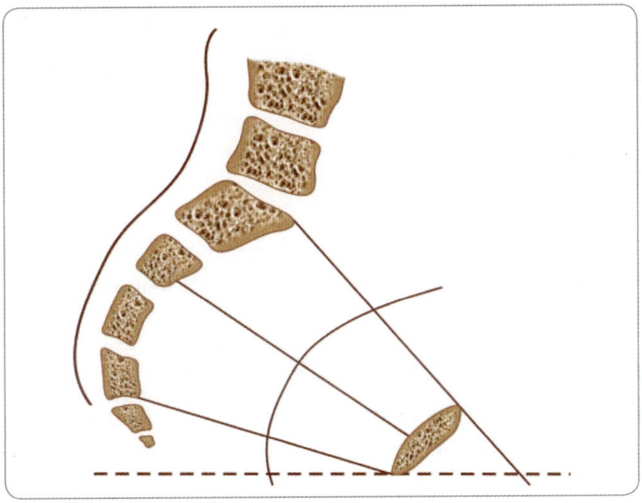

Fig. 3: Pelvic axis – this imaginary line passes through the mid points of the anteroposterior diameters of the pelvis

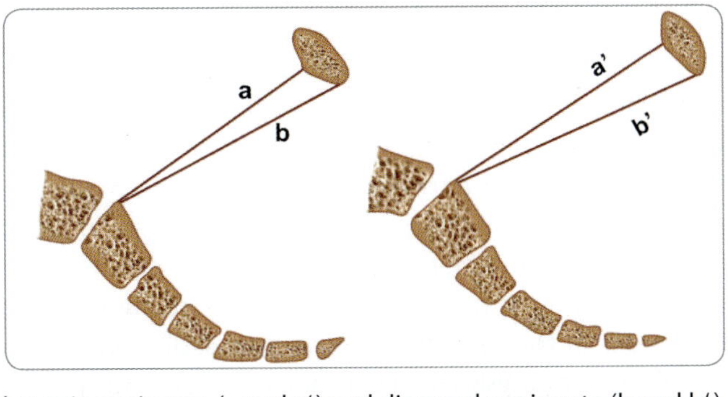

Fig. 4: Obstetric conjugate (a and a') and diagonal conjugate (b and b'). Note the shape and inclination of the symphysis pubis alter the diameter

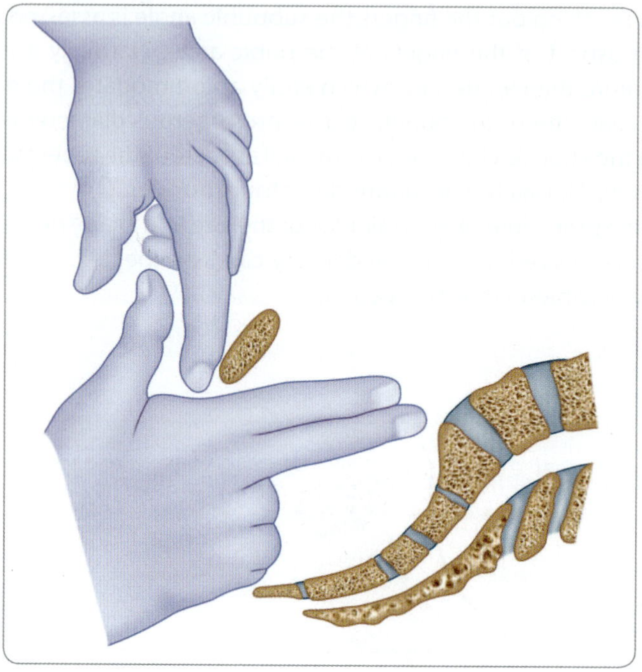

Fig. 5: Pelvic assessment – measurement of the diagonal conjugate

❒ CEPHALOPELVIC DISPROPORTION

Cephalopelvic disproportion means disparity between the size of the fetal head and the capacity of the pelvis. Disproportion may result in a contracted pelvis with an average-sized baby or with a normal pelvis with an over-sized baby.

While assessing the capacity attempts should be made to exclude possible cephalopelvic disproportion. The tips of the examining fingers are placed at the level of the ischial spine and with the left hand the fetal head is grasped gently. As the lower segment of the uterus is almost always tender one should be very gentle while grapsing the head. Then the fetal head is pushed downward and backward (i.e. along the axis of the pelvis). If there is no disproportion at the brim the fetal head can be made to engage and the lower bony point of the head can be felt by the vaginal fingers. The degree of disproportion, if any, can be assessed by putting the thumb of the examining hand over the pubic symphysis. The three degrees of cephalopelvic disproportion are described as mild, moderate and severe. When the head cannot be pushed in, the thumb over the symphysis pubis is used to determine the relation of the fetal head to the upper border of the symphysis. If the fetal skull bone is flushed to the upper border of the symphysis the disproportion is of moderate degree. If the

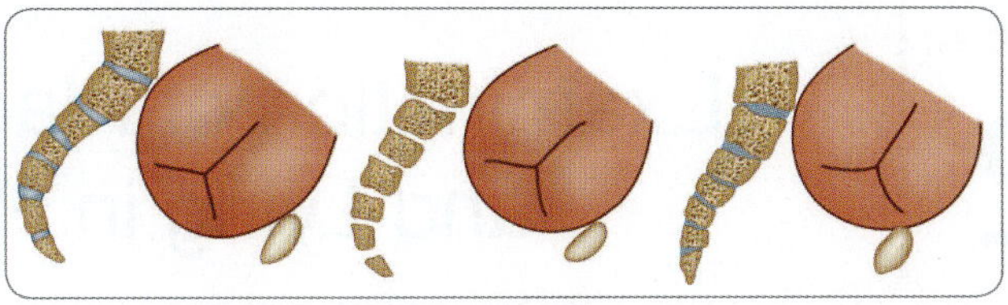

Fig. 6: Assessment of cephalopelvic disproportion – Munro Kerr's method

skull bone overhangs the symphysis, there is a major degree of cephalopelvic disproportion. In mild degree skull is not flushed but the head cannot be pushed into the pelvic.

Sometimes, of course, even though there is no disproportion the head cannot be pushed in. That might be due to high station of the fetal head or due to deflexion of the head. In such cases reassessment is done early in labor to exclude cephalopelvic disproportion and decision is taken as to the mode of delivery.

chapter

12 Examination of Placenta and Lying in Period

After delivery of the fetus, the uterus becomes smaller in size with the placenta still inside. The uterus is almost pyriform in shape and the fundus lies below the level of the umbilicus with the lower pole inside the pelvic cavity. At this stage the uterus is less mobile from side to side.

Following separation from the uterine wall, the placenta gradually comes down to lie in the vagina and so there is apparent lengthening of the umbilical cord still attached to the placenta. The signs of separation of the placenta are the apparent lengthening of the umbilical cord, the uterus becomes smaller and hard, globular in shape and more mobile.

When the placenta is expelled it should be carefully held in hand and with gentle traction the membranes are taken out. It is easy to strip off the membranes from the uterine wall by rotating the placenta. The duration of third stage of labor varies from 15 minutes to 1 hour.

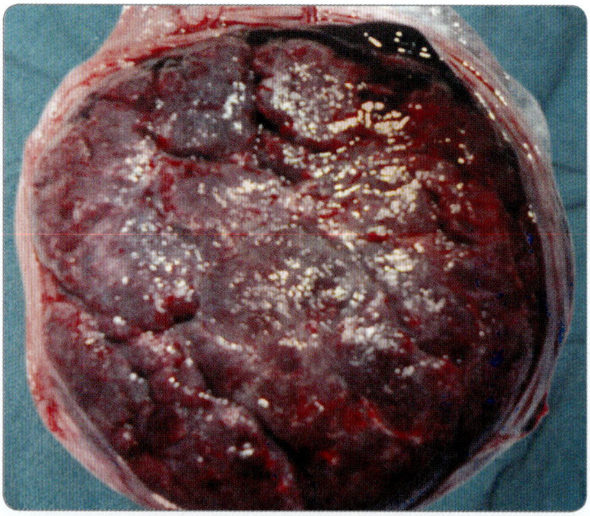

Fig. 1: Maternal surface of normal placenta

❒ EXAMINATION OF PLACENTA

The placenta and membranes after expulsion should be examined carefully. The first thing to notice is whether the placenta and membranes are expelled completely or not. For this purpose the placenta is held on the palms of both hands held together. The maternal surface is exposed removing the covering membranes and examined whether there is any gap. If there is no gap the placenta is completely separated (Fig. 3).

Next is to look for the presence of succenturiate lobe. A succenturiate lobe may be developed away from the main mass of placenta and big vessels run from the main mass along the membranes to that lobe (Fig. 5). In case such a lobe is retained a hole is seen in the membranes and torn vessels are seen. Any other abnormality of the placenta is noted. Then the placenta is weighed and weight is noted.

Membranes are also examined to ensure complete expulsion. Placenta is held by the cord and allowed to hang. In this way the membranes can be examined fully (Fig. 4).

❒ LYING IN PERIOD

After delivery of the child and placenta reproductive organs gradually return back to its pre-pregnant state. This period is known as puerperium. The time taken for this return is about 6 weeks. Another important event after delivery, at least for the mother, is the arrival of a new baby and subsequently onset of lactation.

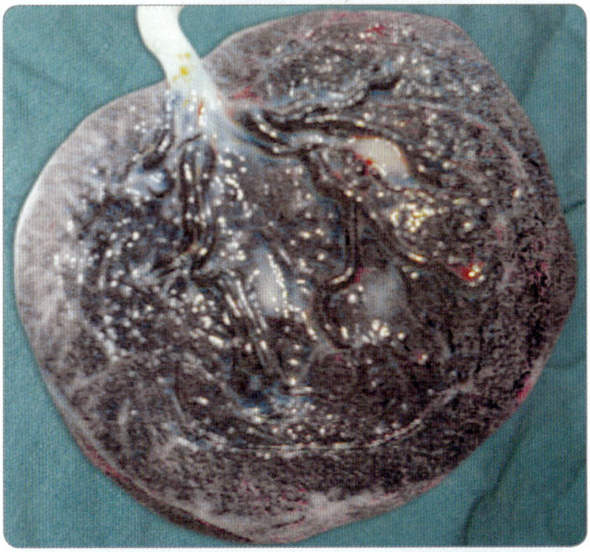

Fig. 2: Fetal surface of normal placenta

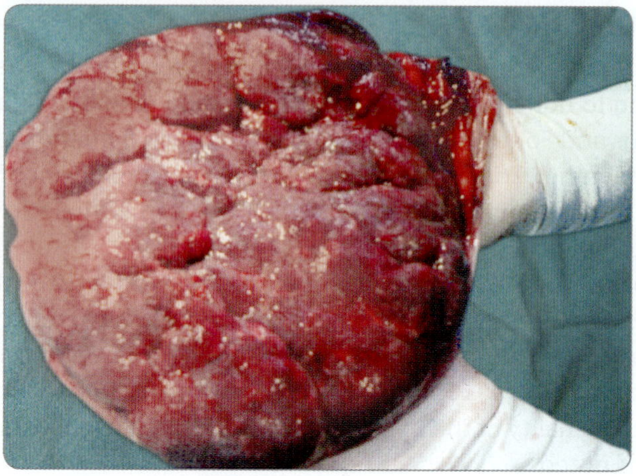

Fig. 3: Examination of placenta after expulsion

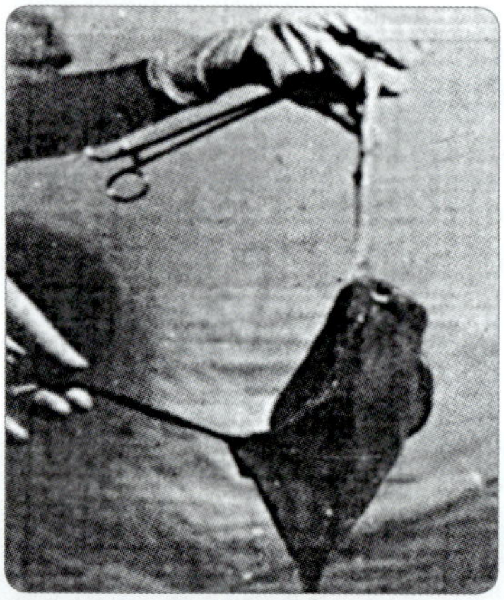

Fig. 4: Examination of membranes

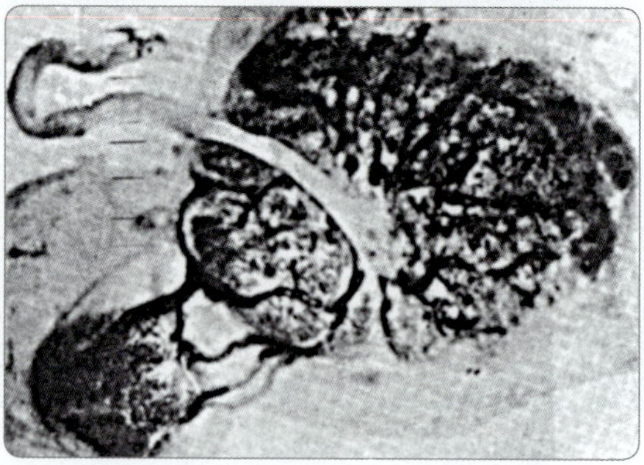

Fig. 5: Placenta succenturiata. (Note the vessels running from the main mass of placenta)

After labor the uterus is a thick muscular organ weighting about 1 kg. Retraction of the uterine musculature and diminished vascular supply help in autolysis, a process by which the size of the uterus is reduced. By 10th day postpartum, the uterus becomes a pelvic organ and is no longer palpable per abdomen.

The torn sinuses of the placental site becomes thrombosed and the area remains ragged with parts of spongy layer of decidua and torn ends of the endometrial glands. The degenerated superficial layer of endometrium is cast off. New epithelium regenerates from the remains of stromal tissue and from the torn end of the endometrial glands.

Along with the uterus other pelvic structures also undergo involution. The vagina, pelvic musculature and ligaments regain their tone, but some amount of laxity still remains. That is a permanent state.

❒ LOCHIA

The vaginal discharge during puerperium is lochia. The superficial necrotic layer of the endometrium is cast off with lochia. So the lochia contains erythrocytes, leukocytes and cast off bits of decidua. For the first few days it contains blood so that color is red and is called "lochia rubra". Lochia rubra continues for 3–4 days, then gradually it becomes paler and is called "lochia serosa". After 10 days lochia is almost yellowish-white or white, called "lochia alba".

During the first few days after delivery the woman should be observed for any new development. After labor pulse, blood pressure and temperature are recorded. There might be slight rise of temperature which is normal. When a hand is placed over the uterus its rhythmic contraction can be felt. A careful assessment is made of any abnormal vaginal bleeding. The size of the uterus may increase and the uterus may be flabby when blood is collected inside it. In this condition there may be only small amount of vaginal bleeding or there may not be at all.

❒ PULSE AND TEMPERATURE

Pulse and temperature should be recorded, if possible, every 4–6 hourly. There should not be any rise of pulse rate or temperature. Temperature of 98.4°F or more is regarded as abnormal.

❒ HEIGHT OF THE FUNDUS

The rate of decrease in fundal height is half an inch everyday. The symphysis-fundal height is measured with a measuring tape everyday at a fixed time after evacuation of bowel and bladder. This simple procedure gives an idea whether the rate of involution is normal or there is subinvolution. By 10th day postpartum fundus lies at the level of the symphysis pubis.

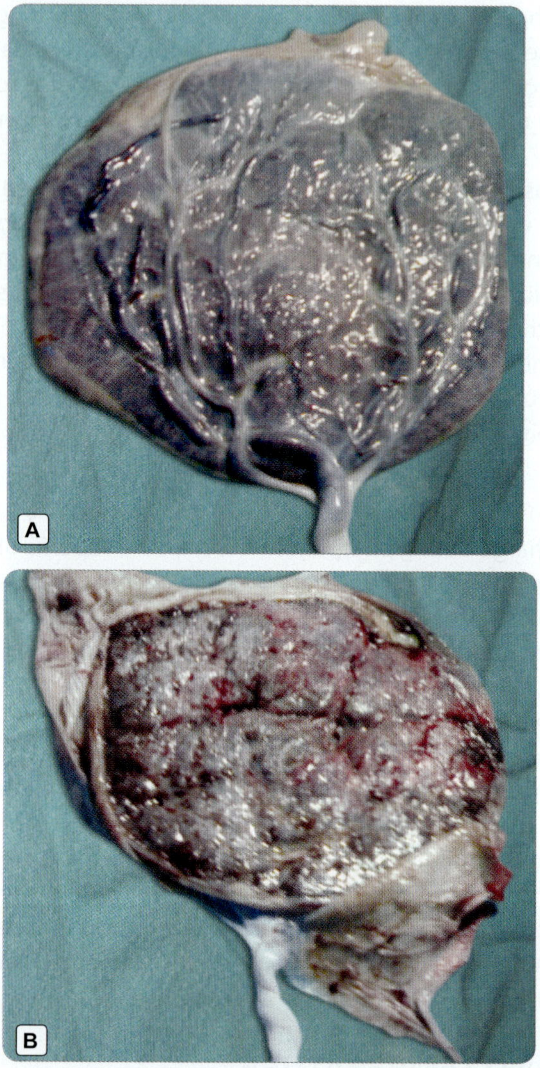

Figs 6A and B: Battledore Placenta – (A) Fetal surface, (B) Maternal surface. (Note the marginal attachment of the umbilical cord)

❐ EXAMINATION OF LOCHIA

Lochia is examined for color and amount. Lochia is red in color for a few days only. In case of persistence of red lochia sub-involution or infection or retained placental tissue should be suspected. Excessive lochia is also abnormal. Foul smelling lochia might be there even without actual genital tract infection. However, when lochia is foul smelling infection should be excluded.

❒ BREAST

During early puerperiun mother is asked about any difficulty in breast or breast feeding. Every mother should be encouraged for breast feeding. On 3rd or 4th day postpartum when there is secretion of milk , efforts should be made to avoid breast engorgement. If engorgement starts breasts become firm and tender and there may be rise of temperature.

❒ BLADDER FUNCTION

The women is asked about her bladder function. Sometimes there may be urinary retention even though the woman may not feel it. A full bladder

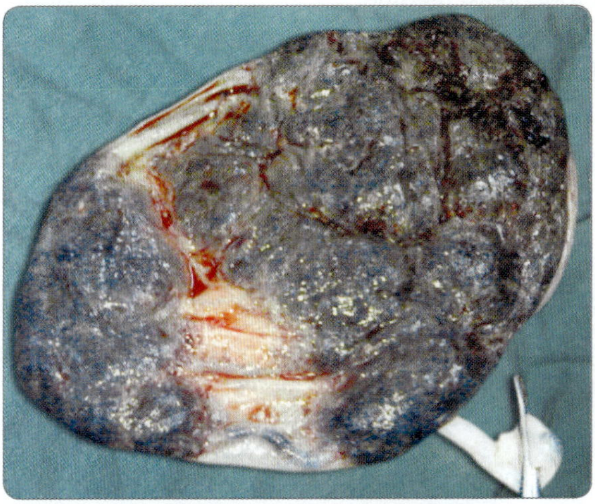

Fig. 7: Bilobed placenta

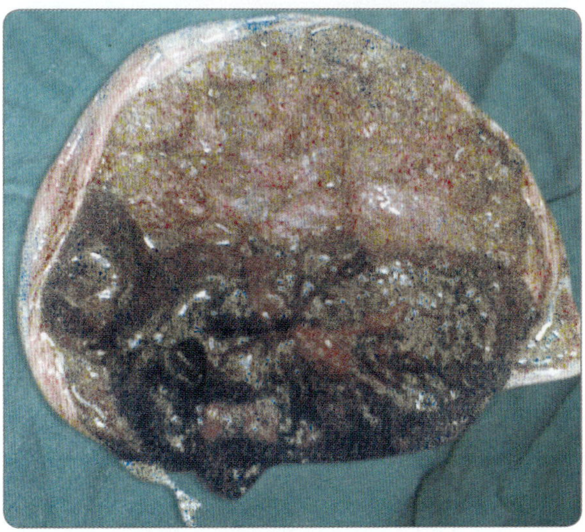

Fig. 8: Accidental hemorrhage

displaces the uterus upward and the bladder can be felt suprapubically. Reflex for micturation may be inhibited by perineal tear or painful episiotomy stitches. Sometimes, of course, atony of bladder musculature may lead to urinary retention.

❐ EXAMINATION OF VULVA AND PERINEUM

Vulva and perineum are examined for signs of hematoma formation in those cases where episiotomy is done during delivery.

Before discharge from hospital the woman should be examined thoroughly in respect of her general condition, involution of uterus, condition of cervix, vagina and vulva. Special attention is paid to the examination of breasts and ensure satisfactory breast feeding.

❐ POSTNATAL EXAMINATION

It is usual practice to ask the woman to report for postnatal examination six weeks after delivery. During the postnatal visit the woman is asked about her general health and health of the baby, breast feeding and whether she has any difficulties.

❐ GENERAL HEALTH

Enquiry is made about her general well-being, diet, rest and bowel habit. She is asked if she has urinary complaints.

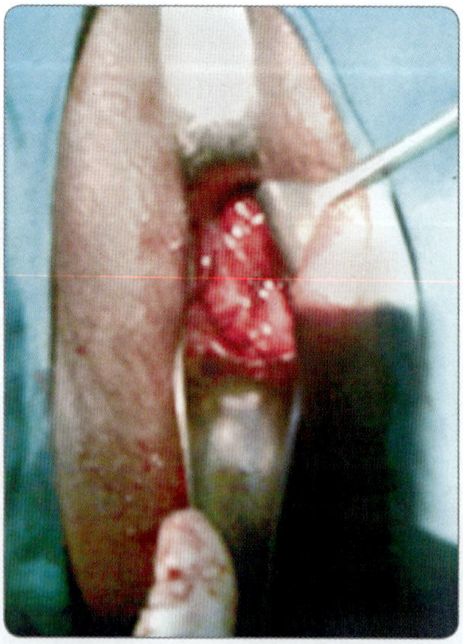

Fig. 9: The cervix after delivery

❐ GENERAL EXAMINATION

In general examination special attention is paid to pulse, blood pressure, and pallor. For those women who had hypertension during pregnancy recording of blood pressure during postnatal check up is important. If hypertension persists further investigations are advised. Anemia among the women in our country is very common and efforts should be made to detect anemia and if present, degree of anaemia is determined and treated accordingly.

❐ SYSTEMIC EXAMINATION

Systemic examination is carried out in usual manner. Abdominal examination is performed and any undue tenderness in lower abdomen is elicited. Tenderness in lower abdomen points to presence of some residual infection.

❐ PELVIC EXAMINATION

Inspection: Vulva and perineum are examined to exclude presence of perineal tear and to note the state of episiotomy wound.

Vagina is examined to detect residual laxity or associated cystocele and rectocele. The most important part of this examination is inspection of the cervix. For this purpose a vaginal speculum is introduced gently and cervix is exposed. Cervix is inspected to detect cervical erosion or cervical tear or ectropion. If the cervix looks unhealthy a smear is taken and sent to laboratory for cytological examination.

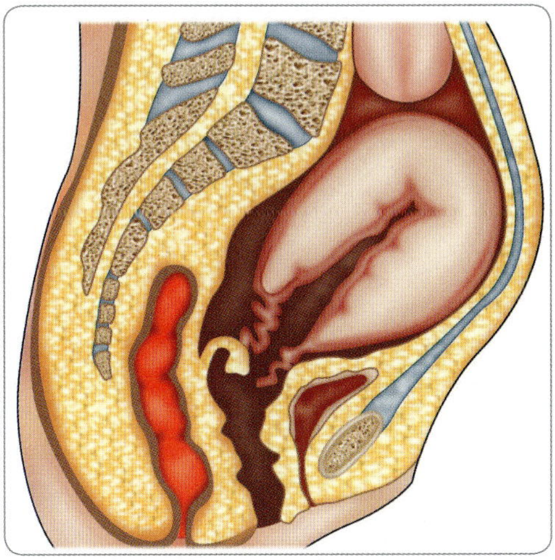

Fig. 10: The uterus after delivery

❐ BIMANUAL EXAMINATION

Bimanual examination is performed to assess the size and position of the uterus, its mobility and to elicit tenderness, if any, in pelvis. Presence of tenderness indicates residual pelvic infection. Next, the laxity of the pelvic floor is assessed and presence of descent of the uterus and/or of the vaginal walls are noted.

This is the appropriate time to review the course and outcome of the last pregnancy. Medical disorders like hypertension, diabetes mellitus, anemia complicating last pregnancy can be reviewed and if needed help of physician is sought for. This is the time the couple is advised for appropriate contraceptive measures, regarding the type of contraceptive suitable for her and the time since when she is to start it.

chapter

13 Assessment of Fetal Well Being

The aim of antenatal assessment of fetal condition is to identify the fetus at increased risk of intrauterine hypoxia and ultimately of fetal death. Recent years have witnessed a great expansion of knowledge of the human fetus and its intrauterine environment. Fetal medicine has established itself as a clinical discipline with great potentiality for favorably influencing the quality of human offspring. The fetus has now achieved the status of a "second patient."

Different tests have been developed to evaluate the well being of different systems of the fetus. Of course, there is a need for a careful and co-ordinated interpretation of the findings of these tests before any action is planned.

It is now possible not only to identify, but to quantify with some precision, physical abnormalities and functional derangement.

That affects the fetus. In some instances, treatment surgical as well as medical can be implemented while the fetus is in uterus. Moreover, accurate dating of gestational age and prediction of lung maturity have enabled the obstetrician to proceed for intervention whenever indicated.

❐ FETAL MOVEMENT IN INTRAUTERINE LIFE

With ultrasonography, movement of the human embryo can be recognized as early as the seventh post-menstrual week. As embryonic and fetal neurological development progress the character of activities changes. From the middle of second trimester mother can appreciate fetal activity. The number of movements perceived by the mother during the day is subjected to wide variation. It is observed that fetal activity diminishes over a period of several days and the movement ceases altogether between 12–48 hours before actual fetal death occurs from asphyxia.

Appreciation of fetal activity by the mother is utilized to assess the fetal state in uterus by the mother herself. This may reduce fetal demise caused by asphyxia. The mother is able to appreciate about 70–80 percent of gross fetal movement. Generally from 32 weeks onwards the number of fetal movement gradually decreases, but remains almost constant at 10 movements in 12 hours period. This is taken as lower limit of normal for clinical purpose.

❐ FACTORS AFFECTING INTRAUTERINE FETAL ACTIVITY

Both maternal and fetal factors may influence the activity of the fetus in intrauterine life.

Maternal factors are maternal activity, obesity and medications to the mother.

Fetal factors are anterior position of the placenta, hydramnios and fetal anomaly.

Appreciation of fetal movement by the mother is very subjective. Some women fail to appreciate even gross fetal movement, on the other hand some women count several movements. Generally, they are less aware of fetal movement when they are busy in their household works or in office works. However, a fetus may remain inactive during intrauterine sleep. Fetus of sedated mother is also sedated and may exhibit less activity. Again another maternal factor influencing appreciation of fetal movement is obesity. These are the difficulties with fetal movement monitoring. But it is a non-invasive test of fetal well-being by which the pregnant women can monitor her fetus herself. It is useful in screening intrauterine fetal activity.

Several methods are described to monitor fetal activity by the mother. The ideal method is thought to be the Cardiff `count to ten' method. In this method a chart has been devised for the mother to plot fetal movement. The chart begins at 9 AM and continues in half-hourly blocks of time until 3 PM. The women counts the fetal movement till the tenth movement is felt and fill in the half-hour block of time in which tenth movement falls. In an active baby ten movements are felt early in the day whereas in a sluggish baby it is delayed.

In another more simplified procedure the mother is advised to count fetal movement for one hour each in the morning, at mid-day and in the evening. The total number of movements felt during these 3 hours time are multiplied by 4 to get a movement count for 12 hours. Total movement during these 12-hour period should be 10–12. If the number of movement is less than 10, further evaluation of the fetus is advised.

Who Needs Antepartum Fetal Monitoring?

Maternal complications which may lead to utero placental insufficiency resulting in fetal hypoxia and eventually intrauterine fetal death need ante partum monitoring. These mothers should be put to adequate fetal monitoring. Following are the maternal complications that may cause utero placental insufficiency:

- When the age of the mother is more
- Pregnancy with history of previous stillbirth
- Suspected IUGR
- Multiple pregnancy
- Prolonged pregnancy
- Oligo hydramnios
- Maternal medical complications such as hypertensive disorder of pregnancy
- Diabetes mellitus
- Chronic renal disease, etc.

Besides these conditions routine fetal monitoring should be advised to all pregnant women. For routine purpose simple clinical monitoring and daily fetal movement count (DFMC) may be sufficient. Once the mother complains of less fetal movement further evaluation is needed to exclude fetal hypoxia. In a fetus of normal growth pattern, and without any maternal risk factor external manipulation may elicit fetal movement and that is what is needed. If the fetus is having IUGR or some maternal risk factors are present cardiotocography is helpful to exclude fetal asphyxia.

❑ CLINICAL ASSESSMENT

The first step in the assessment of the fetus at risk is a careful review of the mother's family history, medical and social history. Details of past obstetric history regarding any complications during the previous pregnancy should be noted. The condition of the baby during previous delivery should be enquired, particularly whether any baby was growth restricted or hypoxic at birth.

It is of vital importance to assess the gestational age correctly. Inaccurate gestational age is confirmed by ultrasonic scan in early pregnancy, if it is doubtful following a careful menstrual history and pelvic examination.

In each subsequent visit gestational age should be confirmed along with examination for lie, presentation, etc. Assessment of the fundal height in relation to the level of the umbilicus is found to be erroneous. It is better to measure the height of the fundus from symphysis pubis with the help of a measuring tape and expressed in centimeter. Amount of liquor amnii present is a useful guide to assess the duration of pregnancy.

Symphysis Fundal Height Measurement

Serial measurement of the symphysis fundal height and girth of the abdomen is an important screening test for detection of intrauterine growth restriction.

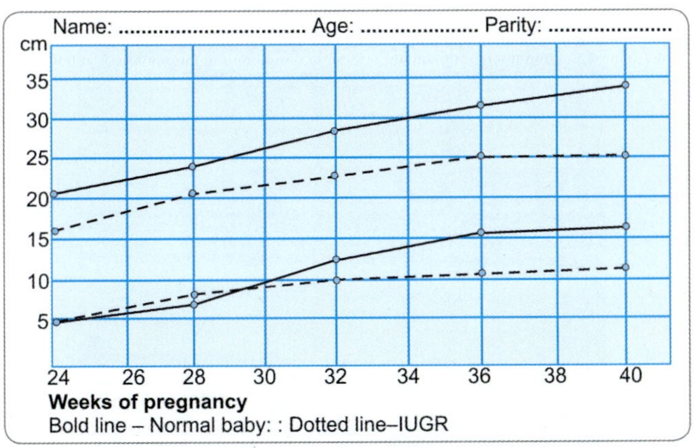

Fig. 1: Curve showing increase in symphysis – fundal height and increase in abdominal girth

Measurement is taken from the symphysis pubis to the top of the fundus with a measuring tape calibrated in centimeter chapter 8 (Figs 2A and B). In the third trimester this measurement equals the gestational age in weeks. Along with

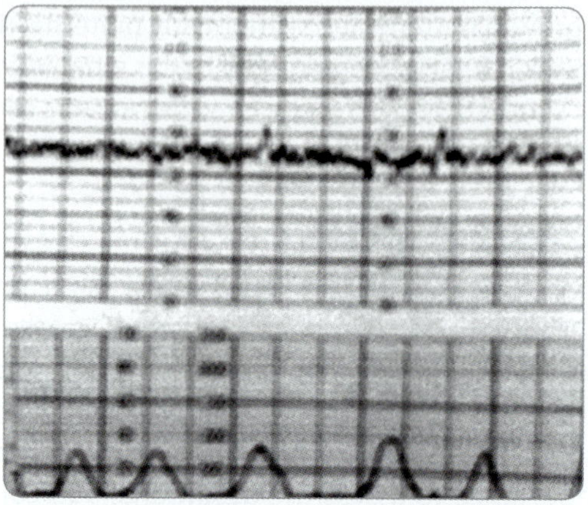

Fig. 2: Fetal heart variability

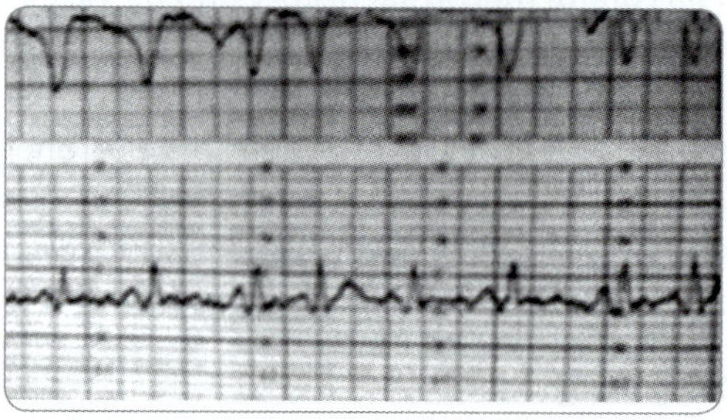

Fig. 3: Early deceleration

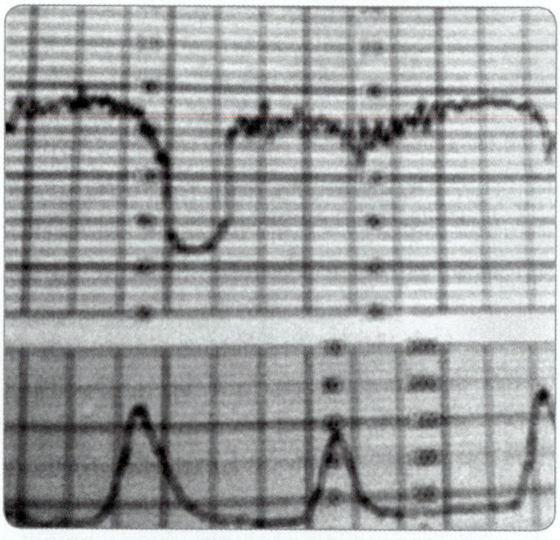

Fig. 4: Late deceleration

the symphysis fundal height, girth of the abdomen at the level of the umbilicus should be taken at each visit. In a normally growing fetus these measurements show gradual increment. Failure to grow or if the fundal height is less than expected for that gestational age further investigations are recommended.

❒ CARDIOTOCOGRAPHY

Cardiotocography (CTG) is a means to monitor fetal heart rate variations over time along with the effect of uterine activity on fetal heart rate. In ante natal period normal CTG shows a baseline rate of 110–150 beats per minute with variability of 5–25 beats per minute. There should be at least two acceleration within every 20 minutes and there should be no deceleration.

An abnormal CTG shows baseline upto 10 beats per minute outside the normal, variability less than 5 beats per minute without acceleration or with deceleration. But it should be remembered that some abnormal pattern may be shown during cyclical fetal inactivity which may return to normal when fetus again becomes active. This period of reduced activity may be of about 20–30 minutes.

If the abnormality persists further evaluation is warranted. CTG is useful method to exclude fetal hypoxia. It can be employed if the mother complains of less fetal movement and in pregnancy with maternal complications which may lead to uteroplacental insufficiency and fetal hypoxia.

Triple Test

Triple test refers to estimation of three maternal biochemical parameters in blood as maternal serum alpha fetoprotein (MSAFP), unconjugated estriol and β-human chorionic gonadotropin (β-hCG) at around 16 weeks of gestation. Down syndrome is a common chromosomal anomaly in which triple test is done as a screening procedure. In Down syndrome the serum level of MSAFP and that of estriol is lower than in mothers with a normal fetus. Whereas β-HCG level is raised than in normal for the corresponding period of gestation.

Besides neural tube defects raised MSAFP may be associated with poor obstetric outcome, particularly IUGR, increased perinatal mortality, pre-eclampsia. Raised level may be due to abdominal wall defect, congenital nephrosis, proximal bowel obstruction of fetus, etc.

Biochemical Test

In intrauterine life the fetus and the placenta are together referred to as 'feto-placental unit'. Various hormones and enzymes were estimated in the past to monitor the functions of feto-placental unit. The widely estimated biochemical parameters include:

1. Steroid hormone – estrogen
2. Human placental lactogen

3. Enzymes – alkaline phosphate
4. Human chorionic gonadotropin
5. Alpha fetoprotein

Estrogens

Estriol output in the maternal urine depends upon integrity of each part of the biosynthetic chain and reduction in secretion does not necessarily indicate placental dysfunction. Conditions like anencephaly with failure of pituitary development, congenital adrenal hypoplasia, congenital cirrhosis and placental sulfatase deficiency result in a fall in maternal estriol output.

Single urinary estriol value is of limited value in assessing fetal status, only repeated tests determining the trend of values are of major importance.

Human Placental Lactogen

Human placental lactogen (HPL) is secreted by the placenta. It is also known as human chorionic somatomammotropin. Sequential determination of HPL in cases of threatened abortion is useful to know the status of the pregnancy. In later weeks of pregnancy measurements seem to offer a means of predicting unexpected fetal distress during labor.

Enzymes

Placenta secretes various enzymes. Serum alkaline phosphatase is one of such enzyme. Measurement of serum alkaline phosphates (heat stable) has been used as an index of the placental isoenzymes. Unfortunately this offers little information as to possible IUGR and compares unfavorably with other parameters.

As these are poor predictor of fetal well-being these are no longer advocated for clinical use.

Human Chorionic Gonadotropin (hCG)

It is also secreted by the placenta and its production is maximum in the first trimester. Measurement of hCG level in late pregnancy for determination of fetal status is of little value. Whereas high level in early pregnancy is useful in the diagnosis and follow-up of hydatidiform mole.

Alpha Fetoprotein

It is an important protein in early weeks of gestation. Most of it is produced by the fetal liver. Alpha fetoprotein (AFP) attains its highest concentration in fetal serum at 12th week of intrauterine life. Thereafter concentration declines slowly until term.

It has been estimated that routine screening of maternal blood samples around 16–20 weeks of gestation can detect 20 percent of affected cases. Moreover, in late pregnancy any condition causing fetal distress may lead to increase of AFP in maternal serum.

Ultrasonography

Ultrasonography helps the obstetricians in a big way to assess the fetal health in utero. The growth of the fetus is measured by estimation of biparietal diameter, abdominal circumference and femur length. Again fetal well-being can be assessed by fetal biophysical profile.

❐ BIPARIETAL DIAMETER

Biparietal diameter (BPD) of the fetal head has been used for many years to assess the fetal growth. It is the only measurement of the head which can be made independent of the presentation or the degree of flexion of the head. Normally, the ratio of growth of biparietal diameter is 3.5 mm per week between 16 and 26 weeks and 2 mm per week between 26 and 36 weeks of gestation. To have a correct picture of the growth pattern a serial study of BPD is essential. It is difficult to determine from an isolated measurement taken in third trimester whether the given fetus is small for date or not.

❐ ABDOMINAL CIRCUMFERENCE

Measurement of abdominal circumference (AC) is another important parameter. Early evidence of intrauterine growth restriction can be obtained by comparing head and abdominal size. When fetal abdomen is small but BPD is more or less appropriate for gestational age asymmetrical IUGR can be concluded. When both BPD and abdominal circumference are small wrong date is a possibility. The ratio of BPD and abdominal circumference is a sensitive measurement when plotted against gestational age.

Fetal weight can be estimated by ultrasonography. But the error is higher (8–10%).

❐ FETAL BIOPHYSICAL PROFILE

Fetal biophysical activities directly reflect the function of fetal central nervous system. Fetal nervous system regulates the various dynamic biophysical varieties such as breathing movement, heart rate, reactivity, tone, etc. Central nervous system is highly sensitive to oxygen concentration of blood. So a given variable is an indirect evidence of degree of oxygenation of the central nervous system. Various variables are defined, redefined and modified. At present the following are taken into account:

a. Fetal breathing movement (FBM)
b. Gross body movement (GBM)
c. Fetal tone (FT)
d. Qualitative amniotic fluid volume (AFV).

Fetal Breathing Movement

In healthy human fetus breathing movement can be observed. These breathing movements are regulated by CNS. The proportion of time spent in breathing varies with the time of day, reaching its zenith in late evening. Fetal hypoxemia and/or acidemia produces prolonged fetal apnea. Clinical data suggests a definite relationship between the presence or absence of fetal breathing movement and condition of the fetus at birth. There should be at least 1 episode of FBM of 30 seconds in 30 minutes.

Gross Body Movement

Maternal perception of fetal movement is an easily available fetal biophysical activity. But the mother may not feel the smaller movements. In such situation ultrasound allows a more accurate appraisal of fetal movement. The greatest number of movements may be observed in the fetal limbs, but these are of short duration and only accounts for a small percentage of movements. Major movements involving all four fetal parts under observation account for a major percentage of movements. A suggested norm is at least 3 discrete body/limb movements in 30 minutes.

Fetal Tone

Normal fetal tone is defined as prompt return to flexion after extension of the limbs or trunk. Fetal tone is defined as abnormal when either fetal movements are not associated with return to position of flexion or when fetal movements are absent and the fetus is in a complete or partial deflexed position with fetal hands open.

Amniotic Fluid Volume

Amount of liquor amnii is said to be adequate when 1 or more than 1 cm or longer pockets of fluid is detected in two perpendicular planes. Oligohydramnios may reflect IUGR.

❐ ELECTRONIC FETAL MONITORING

Electronic fetal heart monitoring is a popular technique in developed countries. In our country these sophisticated equipments are not readily available and is only available in few selected centers. External fetal heart monitoring is used during pregnancy. Two methods are available – non-stress and contraction stress tests.

❐ NON-STRESS TEST

It is often used as a screening test. The rationale of the test is that acceleration of fetal heart rate in association with fetal movement indicates an intact and responsive central nervous system. Fetuses showing this response are said to be `reactive' and those not responding are termed `non-reactive'.

❐ CONTRACTION STRESS TEST

The idea of contraction stress test is to study the response of fetal heart rate pattern to uterine contraction. But it is an invasive technique and initiates labor and may be hazardous to an already compromised fetus. For these difficulties this technique is not favored nowadays.

❐ AMNIOCENTESIS

Examination of the amniotic fluid provides some important information regarding the state of the fetus in utero. Aspiration of a sample of amniotic fluid provides for a variety of diagnostic tests.

❐ ASSESSMENT OF LUNG MATURITY

Maturity of lung is of importance for survival of the newborn. It is essential that lung alveoli are maintained at a state of expansion to prevent alveolar collapse in expiration. This important function is attributed to a lipoprotein called surfactant.

The surface active phospholipids are synthesized by the epithelium of the lung alveoli—the pneumocytes. Among different phospholipids lecithin (phosphatidyl cholines) comprises maximum amount. So the relative concentration of lecithin to sphingomyelin (L/S ratio) in amniotic fluid is considered as a sensitive index of lung maturity.

It is estimated that when the lecithin/sphingomyelin ratio (L/S ratio) is greater than 2, the risk of developing respiratory distress is low and if the ratio is less than 2 the risk is more. In clinical practice the test can be performed in a simple way.

❐ FOAM STABILITY TEST (SHAKE TEST)

The principle of foam stability test or shake test is that when amniotic fluid containing surfactant is mixed with appropriate amount of ethanol, stable foam is formed at the air-liquid interface. This is an easy and quick test. In a clean glass tube 1 mL of recently collected amniotic fluid is added to 1 mL of 95 percent ethanol. Into another tube 0.5 mL of amniotic fluid is added to 0.5 mL of normal saline and 1 mL of 95 percent ethanol. Both the tubes are vigorously shaken for 15 seconds and placed upright in a rack for 15 minutes. The presence of an intact ring of bubbles at the air liquid interface after 15 minutes indicates a positive test.

❐ AMNIOTIC FLUID BILIRUBIN

Bilirubin in amniotic fluid is derived from hemolysis of fetal red cells. Normally concentration of bilirubin in amniotic fluid comes down with advancing gestational age and almost negligible at term. But in conditions of increased hemolysis of fetal red blood cells, concentration of bilirubin in amniotic fluid also increases significantly. In Rhesus hemolytic diseases spectrophotometric study of bilirubin is important to evaluate the degree of hemolysis or its effect on the fetus. Estimation of some other constituents of amniotic fluid are suggested to determine the fetal maturity. But most of these constituents reflect the maturity of certain organs only. These include amniotic fluid creatinine concentration, osmolarity of amniotic fluid and concentration of lipid laden cells.

❐ RISK OF AMNIOCENTESIS

Amniocentesis is an invasive technique with some attending risks. These are:

1. Injury to the fetus or placenta
2. It may initiate abortion or premature labor
3. Infection
4. In Rh-negative mother injury to the placenta may enhance maternal isoimmunization and hemolytic disease of the fetus.

Fetal heart activity is controlled by central nervous system. A normal fetal heart sound pattern indirectly signifies adequate oxygenation of the brain tissue. Besides oxygenation or in other words adequate uteroplacental perfusion, there are some other factors which may alter fetal heart rate pattern during labor. These are pressure over the head or the umbilical cord or pressure over the face or neck

❐ INTRAPARTUM MONITORING

The most crucial time for the fetus in utero is during labor. Fetal hypoxia may result any time during labor. If the state of severe hypoxia persists for a long time it may result in intrapartum or early neonatal death. The idea of intrapartum fetal monitoring is to detect fetal hypoxia at an early stage so that if necessary appropriate steps can be undertaken before permanent damage to the fetal brain takes place.

Methods of Intrapartum Monitoring

The methods of intrapartum monitoring are non-invasive and invasive.

Non-invasive methods include:

1. Intermittent auscultation with stethoscope
2. External electronic fetal heart monitoring.

Invasive methods include:

1. Internal fetal heart monitoring
2. Fetal blood sampling.

Intermittent auscultation of fetal heart during labor is an acceptable method to assess the fetal condition. In women with low risk of developing fetal distress during labor this is an effective method. In this method FHR is auscultated every 15 minutes in the first stage and every 5 minutes in the second stage of labor immediately after an uterine contraction.

FHR drops during the height of uterine contraction and recovers promptly as the contraction ends. Fetal heart rate may be determined by using the Doppler instrument also.

External Electronic Monitoring

In this method uterine activity is measured by placing external tocodynamometer on the anterior abdominal wall. The fetal heart rate is also detected through the maternal abdominal wall. To detect fetal heart sound the ultrasound Doppler principle is usually used. Fetal electrocardiogram may be used with the help of electrodes attached to maternal abdomen. Uterine contraction and fetal heart activity are recorded simultaneously and continuously on a moving paper.

Internal Monitoring of Fetal Heart

In this method spiral electrodes are applied to the fetal scalp after rupturing the membranes. To record uterine contraction a small nylon catheter with multiple hole near the tip is connected to a strain gauge transducer to record intrauterine pressure. Fetal heart rate and uterine contractions are recorded continuously on a moving strip of paper.

Fetal Heart Rate Pattern

During labor there should not be any change in fetal heart rate pattern. But very often it shows periodic variation. There might be tachycardia or bradycardia. Following are the different patterns which are described:

Baseline Fetal Heart Rate

Baseline fetal heart rate is recorded between two uterine contractions. A rate of 120–160 beat per minutes is taken as normal.

Deceleration Pattern

Deceleration means slowing of fetal heart rate. Deceleration may be there in relation to uterine contraction. It may precede uterine contraction (early), it may accompanies (mid) or may outlasts uterine contraction (late). Each of these patterns has different significance.

Early Deceleration

Early deceleration is also referred to as Type-I dip. In this type slowing of fetal heart rate occurs at the onset of uterine contraction. It is due to increased intracranial pressure.

Late Deceleration

Late deceleration is referred to as Type-II dip. In this type slowing of fetal heart rate begins near the height of uterine contractions, the rate is often lowest after the contraction passes off and returns to baseline only before the next contraction starts. It is due to fetal hypoxia consequent to uteroplacental insufficiency.

Variable Deceleration

In this type deceleration occurs without any relation to uterine contraction and the degrees of slowing are different in different deceleration. This type of deceleration is due to cord compression.

Baseline Tachycardia

Baseline tachycardia is one when fetal heart rate is more than 160 beats per minute between two uterine contractions. It may be due to some maternal conditions such as fever, dehydration or excitement or may be due to mild fetal hypoxia.

Baseline Bradycardia

Baseline bradycardia is one when fetal heart rate is less than 120 beats per minute. Mild bradycardia without deceleration may not be of any significance or it may be due to congenital heart disease. However, severe bradycardia often precedes fetal death.

Beat to Beat Variation

Beat to beat variation can be studied in internal electronic monitoring. In a normal fetus in late pregnancy there is variation in fetal heart rate. The time interval between two consecutive fixed points in fetal ECG, the R wave, is not fixed. Loss of beat to beat variation is present when the number of beats per minute varies by less than 5 beats. Loss of beat to beat variation is an important finding indicating fetal hypoxia.

Fetal Blood Sampling

Intrauterine hypoxia leads to fetal acidosis and fall in fetal pH, if the state of acidosis continues it may lead to damage to the central nervous system and shows abnormal fetal ECG. Fetal blood sampling is a method by which fetal acidosis can be confirmed by estimating pH of fetal blood. So for confirmation of acidosis fetal blood sampling is necessary. Method of fetal flood sampling was introduced by Saling in 1964 and it is a safe and simple method.

Technique: Keeping the patient in lithotomy position an amnioscope is introduced through a partially dilated cervix. Membranes should already be ruptured. The amnioscope is gently pressed against the fetal scalp. The area of the scalp is wiped clean with cotton swab. Sprayed with ethyl chloride to induce hyperemia and coated with silicone gel. A stab is made with a miniature-guarded blade. When a drop of blood forms on the surface it is immediately collected in a heparinized capillary tube. The pH is determined quickly.

It is generally agreed that a pH of 7.25 or greater is normal and less than 7.20 is abnormal. When it is between 7.20 and 7.24 a repeat estimation may be indicated.

While assessing the fetal blood pH it should be remembered that fetal pH is influenced by maternal pH level. So a low fetal pH may not always reflect the degree of fetal hypoxia if at the same time mother is also acidotic.

❐ DANGER OF ELECTRONIC FETAL HEART MONITORING AND FETAL SCALP BLOOD SAMPLING

These are invasive techniques and as such inherent with some danger.

Trauma

Injury to the fetal scalp in both these techniques may create problem. The placenta may also be injured inadvertently while introducing the intrauterine catheter.

Infection

Both the mother and the fetus may have infection. There may be infection of the fetal scalp wound being infected by the electrode or following blood sampling. There is an increased risk of intrauterine infection also.

It has been observed that perinatal mortality is lower in those labors monitored continuously with electronic fetal heart monitoring. Ideally all labor should be monitored. But, at present it is used only in high-risk pregnancy cases. A normal fetal heart pattern assures the fetal well-being. In almost all cases. But an abnormal pattern may be there even without fetal distress. So to detect actual fetal distress FBS should be done and fetal pH is measured. Decision to interfere should be adequately supported by FBS findings and other clinical parameters. Abnormal fetal heart pattern is considered as a screening test which should be confirmed by FBS and fetal pH estimation.

It should be emphasized that these are delicate procedures involving use of sophisticated instrument. Sufficient experience is needed to handle them. Moreover, care is needed in interpretation of the findings which should always be corroborated with clinical findings.

chapter 14

The Newborn Immediately After Birth

Transition from intrauterine fetal life to extrauterine independent existence is a crucial one. From a fully dependant comfortable intrauterine atmosphere the baby suddenly emerges into a different world full of various stimuli like cold, heat, air, light, etc. Moreover, after clamping the cord there comes about a dramatic change in homodynamics of the baby. But in spite of all these changes transition from intrauterine life to extrauterine one is quite smooth in most of the newborns. Only 10–15 percent of newborn may requite assistance.

More than half of the infants death occurs in first four weeks of life. Half of these deaths takes place in first week of life due to birth asphyxia, hypothermia and infection. Babies born with a low birth weight (< 2500 g) are at higher risk of dying due to these causes.

The basic requirements of newborn infants are immediate assistance at birth when needed, primarily to establish respiration and subsequent assistance in obtaining adequate nutrition, in maintaining normal body temperature and in avoiding contact with infection.

❒ BASIC CARE OF NEWBORN AT BIRTH

The cord should be clamped as soon the baby is completely delivered. Early clamping is advocated in babies with asphyxia, cord around neck and Rhesus isoimmunization. Milking of cord is hazardous in babies with cardiovascular anomalies, intracranial hemorrhage and maternal fetal blood group incompatibility. Holding of babies in inverted position and slapping over buttock or squeezing the stomach or chest should be avoided.

If the baby's mouth contain thick secretion, meconium or blood these should be sucked in the delivery table itself.

The baby is transferred to a pre-warmed flat surface and immediately dried and covered with dry clothe and kept warm. Most babies would cry lustily and do not need any special care.

❒ APGAR SCORE

Apgar score is evaluation of five factors one minute after birth and then after five minutes to detect improvement. These factors are heart rate per minute, respiration, muscle tone, reflex response and color.

Apgar score

Score	0	1	2
Heart rate	Absent	100	100
Respiration	Absent	Slow, gasping	Good, crying
Muscle tone	Flaccid	Some limb flexion	Active
Reflex Response	Nil	Grimace	Cough, sneeze
Color	Pale blue	Body pink, limb blue	pink

Score 7–10 No depression
4–6 Mild depression
0–3 Severe depression

If the Apgar score is 7–10 the baby needs no resuscitation, when the score is 4–6 baby needs resuscitation and in case it is further low the baby is severely depressed and needs resuscitation, may be including endotracheal intubation and positive pressure ventilation.

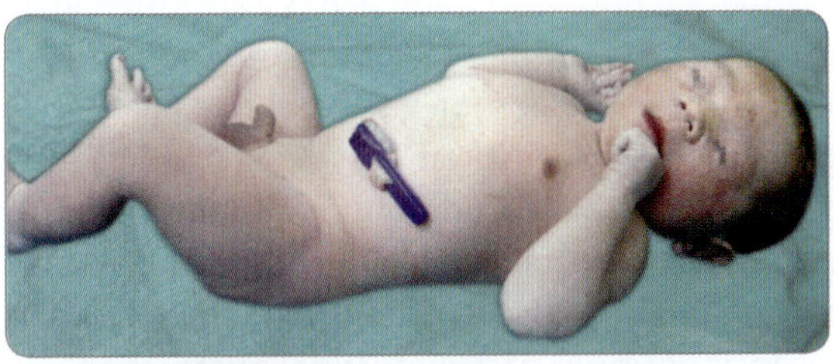

Fig. 1: Mature baby after birth

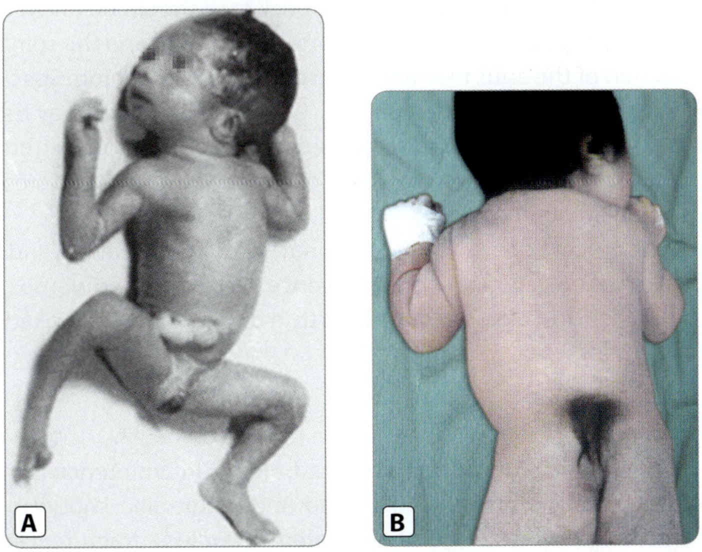

Figs 2A and B: (A) Premature baby (note the vulva with prominent labia minora and clitoris); (B) Term baby with spina bifida – occulta (note the tuft of hair)

Apgar score is a practical method of systematically assisting a newborn baby immediately after birth, to help babies identified requiring resuscitation for hypoxic acidosis. A low Apgar score does not necessarily signify fetal hypoxic acidosis. Additional factors may reduce the score. The Apgar score also does not necessarily predict neonatal morality or subsequent celebral palsy. The one minute Apgar score signals the need for immediate resuscitation and the 5–10–15 minutes Apgar score indicate the probability of successful resuscitation of the baby. Apgar score of 0–3 at 20 minuites signifies high mortality and morbidity.

Although the Apgar score is helpful in evaluating babies in need of attentions, babies who are born limp, cyanotic or apneic require immediate resuscitation prior to assessment of 1 minute Apgar score. Babies with prolapsed cord or delayed delivery with evidence of intrauterine asphyxia should receive prompt resuscitation and close observation subsequently.

After the initial assistance and when the baby is out of danger a thorough examination is carried out. This physical examination is carried out to exclude congenital malformation and birth trauma. It is performed in a systematic way. Examination is started at the head and ends at the toe.

First is inspection of the baby for visible abnormality. Head is examined first. Patency of the nares are ensured passing a small catheter, oral cavity is examined to exclude cleft palate. Then observe the neck for congenital goiter. A feeding tube is passed from the nose, mouth upto the stomach to determine the patency of esophagus and also to note the volume of gastric content which may help in diagnosis of upper gastrointestinal obstruction.

Chest and then abdomen are examined followed by the back. Nipples should be examined. While examining the back care should be taken to ensure whether there is any abnormality of the vertebral column and the spinal cord. A close inspection of the anus may reveal absence of anal opening. Special care is to be taken while examining the genitalia. On rare occasions it may be difficult to assign sex in the newborn and may need further evaluation. Extremities are examined one by one. Fingers should be examined carefully and creases over the sole should be noted.

During the process of examination the nature of cry, urination, and passage of meconium are noted. Skin color, presence of lanugo and vernex caseosa should be looked for. Skin naevi and birth marks should be looked for and presence is noted.

❐ PALPATION

Head is palpated and suture lines are noted. Head circumference is measured with a tape. Any abnormality in the head and suture line should be noted. Clavicle and long bones are gently palpated to exclude fracture. Hip should be examined for undue mobility which may be due to congenital dislocation.

Palpation of the abdomen reveals palpable liver and spleen. Besides these any abnormal lump should be looked for. Auscultation of the chest is important to detect any obstruction to air entry and presence of crepitation. Heart rate and rhythm are noted carefully and pulse of the femoral artery is felt.

❐ REFLEX

Moros reflex is most informative one and should be carried out. It can be elicited by banging the table on which the baby is lying. The baby makes movements of abduction, legs are drawn up and arms are brought together in an embracing manner. This reflex indicates intact neuromuscular co-ordination.

Examination is completed by measuring the length with a measuring tape and taking weight. All these measurements should be noted.

Assessment of Gestational Age After Birth

A careful assessment of the gestational age is done after delivery. Particularly after induction of labor or following elective caesarean section. The aim of this assessment is to find out whether the baby is mature or premature. Preterm and small for date babies are at great risk and need expert pediatric care.

On the basis of gestation age newborn babies are classified as:

Preterm : Babies born before 37 completed weeks of pregnancy.
Term : Babies born between 37 and 42 completed weeks of pregnancy.
Post-term : babies born after 42 weeks of pregnancy.

Another classification is based on birth weight of the babies.

Appropriate for Gestational Age (AGA)

In this group the birth weight of the babies falls between 10th and 90th percentile for gestational age.

Small for Gestational Age (SGA) or Small for Date

In this group birth weight of the babies is less than 10th percentile for the gestational age.

Large of Gestation Age

The birth weight of the babies in this group falls over the 90th percentile for the gestational age.

The following criteria are considered while assigning the gestational age to a newborn baby:

1. Skin
2. Lanugo
3. Breast—areola, nodule
4. Sole creases

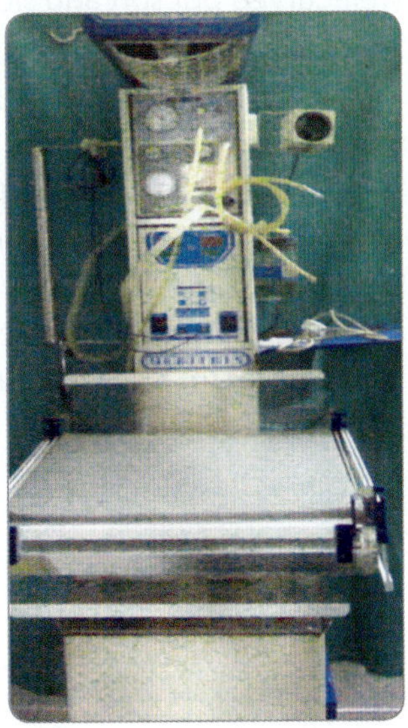

Fig. 3: Baby resuscitation machine

5. Skull firmness
6. Ear
7. Genitalia.

Skin: In a term baby the skin is thick, pale pink, some desquamation is there. In preterm babies the skin is thin, pink, a few vessels may be seen, whereas in post-term babies skin is thick, pale and desquamanting.

Lanugo: In more premature babies lanugo covers the whole body or may be absent over the face. In mature babies lanugo is present over the shoulder, whereas in post-term babies no lanugo is seen.

Breast: Areola of breast is raised in term babies. The nodule measures about 7–10 mm in preterm babies, areola may be apparent or slightly raised and nodule may be 0–3 mm, in post-term babies the areola is raised and the nodule is about 10 mm.

Sole creases: Sole creases are an important sign. In term babies crease involve the heel also, so is in post-term babies with desquamation, whereas in preterm babies there may be no crease or may cover only the anterior half of the sole.

Skulll firmness: Bones are hard but sutures are easy to displace in term babies. In post-term babies bones are hard and suture are difficult to displace, whereas in preterm babies bones are soft particularly at the edges of the fontanelle and sutures are easy to displace.

Ear: Pinas are formed and firm with instant recoil in term babies, in post-term babies ears are stiff with cartilage. But in preterm babies pinas may be flat or well-curved but soft and slow to recoil.

Genitalia: In case of term male babies testes are down with good scrotal rugae. But in preterm babies scrotum may be empty or testes may descend with few rugae.

In female term babies labia majora is large and minora and clitoris are covered. In preterm one majora and minora are equally prominent with prominent clitoris.

Along with the above physical examination neurological examination of the newborn infant is carried out for complete assessment of gestational age of the infant.

chapter 15

Abnormal Presentation and Position

At term in about 96 percent of pregnant women the fetus assumes a longitudinal lie with the cephalic end occupying the lower uterine segment and with flexed attitude. Vertex is the commonest presentation. Rest of the cases have some abnormality in presentation. Near term the fetus has to accomodate itself in the available intrauterine space. In second trimester or in early third trimester the fetus is relatively smaller in size and there remains large amount of liquor amnii inside the uterine cavity. The fetus can move freely and there is no question of adopting a particular position. Later at term the fetus increases in size and amount of liquor amnii reduces making the uterine cavity relatively narrow for the fetus. As a result the fetus has to adopt a position best suited to it. At term pregnancy the uterine cavity is pear-shaped having enough space at the fundus. Towards the end of pregnancy the fetus usually forms an ovoid mass with flexion attitude, where the buttocks with the thighs and legs near it forms a bulky mass (Fig. 1). This bulky mass is easily accomodated at the relatively wide fundal area of the uterine cavity and the head occupies the lower pole of the uterus.

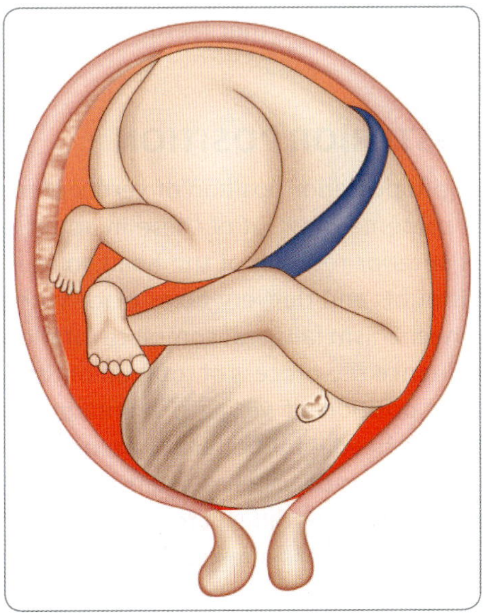

Fig. 1: Fetal ovoid (Note the flexion attitude of the baby)

Few conditions are found to be associated with malpresentation. In premature fetus abnormal presentation is more common because of abundant liquor amnii and relatively bigger size of the head in relation to the trunk. Some fetal abnormalities such as hydrocephalus and anencephaly cause abnormal presentation. In hydrocephalus the big head occupies the fundus of the uterus and the breech is at the lower pole. In anencephaly the vault of the head is absent and face presentation is common. Another important association of malpresentation is multiple pregnancy. Here in this condition owing to non-availability of adequate space the fetus cannot move freely resulting in more malpresentation.

On the other hand in polyhydramnios the fetus can move freely inside the uterine cavity even at term and may lead to malpresentation. In oligohydramnios as the amount of liquor amnii is less than average, fetal movement is restricted causing malpresentation.

Attachment of the placenta in lower uterine segment and contracted pelvis prevent the head from entering the pelvis and lead to oblique or transverse lie. Similarly space occupying lesions in the pelvis such as uterine fibromyoma and ovarian tumor diminishes the available space and cause malpresentation. Uterine anomalies such as bicornuate uterus, septate or subseptate uterus are frequently associated with malpresentation. Association of multiparity with abnormal presentation is likely due to laxity of the anterior abdominal wall musculature, which when normal favors longitudinal lie. Among the other fetal conditions associated with malpresentation are compromised fetus or fetus with decreased activity. Some neurological impairment may be the cause of less fetal activity and fetal malpresentation results owing to less activity. Malpresentation is common with fetal death, again due to absence of fetal activity. Short umbilical cord is another factor which is observed frequently with fetal malpresentation.

❒ OCCIPITOPOSTERIOR POSITION

The incidence of occipitoposterior position of vertex presentation is about 25 percent of all vertex presentation. Out of these in about 80–90 percent there occurs spontaneous anterior rotation of the head so that the occiput comes below the symphysis pubis and delivery takes place without any difficulty. In the rest the normal mechanism fails and complete rotation of the head fails to occur. Few factors influence the process of rotation of the head.

In occipitoposterior position of vertex presentation fetal head is usually deflexed. Deflexion of the head is for better accommodation inside the uterine cavity. The fetal spine which is convex lies against the maternal lumbar spine, which is also convex anteriorly. It is difficult to accomodate two convex surfaces inside the narrow uterine cavity. As a result the fetal spine becomes deflexed. Posterior position of the occiput is usually associated with android type of pelvis, with a narrow anterior segment and wide posterior segment. The wide occiput is well-accommodated in the wide posterior segment of the pelvic inlet. In labor when the head descends through the pelvic inlet the biparietal diameter tends to be held up in the sacro-cotyloid diameter between the sacral promontory and the iliopectineal eminence. The forehead has sufficient space and can descend easily during uterine contraction, increasing degree of deflexion. Further deflexion of the head may lead to even extension of the head causing brow or face presentation.

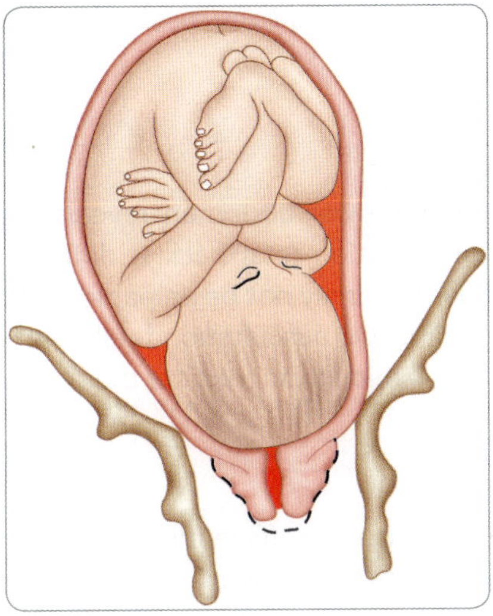

Fig. 2: Occipitoposterior position of vertex presentation

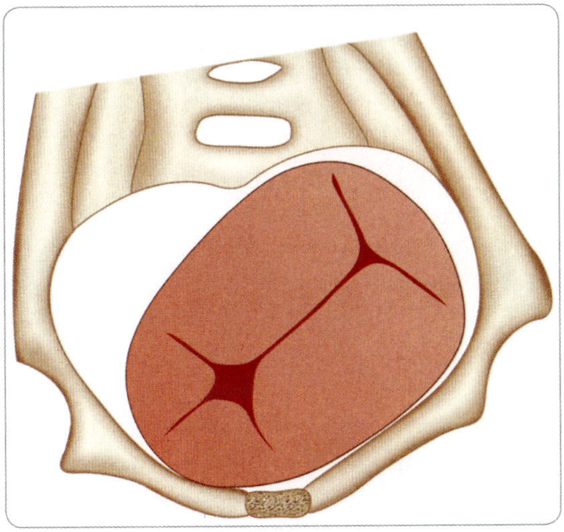

Fig. 3: Occipitoposterior position of vertex presentation (seen from below)

Poor uterine contraction is another factor for non-rotation of the head. Fetal head in a deflexed state does not fit well in the lower uterine segment to initiate good uterine contractions. As a result of weak uterine contraction the head fails to overcome the resistance offered by the pelvic wall. Early rupture of membranes is common with occipitoposterior position. Membranes are ruptured early in labor and almost all the liquor amnii is drained out.

The uterine musculature almost grips the fetal trunk preventing its free movement. Besides these factors which are associated with occipitoposterior position undiagnosed mild cephalopelvic disproportion is one which should be considered.

❒ DIAGNOSIS

Abdominal Examination

Careful observation of the lower abdomen reveals slight flattening of the suprapubic region. On palpation fetal back is difficult to locate. It may be palpable towards the flanks or may not be palpable at all. Fetal limbs are easily felt on both side of midline. On auscultation fetal heart sound may be heard towards the flanks or in the midline. In the later the sound is heard directly over the chest.

Vaginal Examination

In early labor as the cervix is not sufficiently dilated and vertex is high up, it is difficult to diagnose occipitoposterior position by vaginal examination. Moreover, an elongated bag of membranes may bulge and while trying to feel the presenting part it may rupture. It becomes easy to feel the sutures and fontanelle after few hours of labor, when cervix is sufficiently dilated.

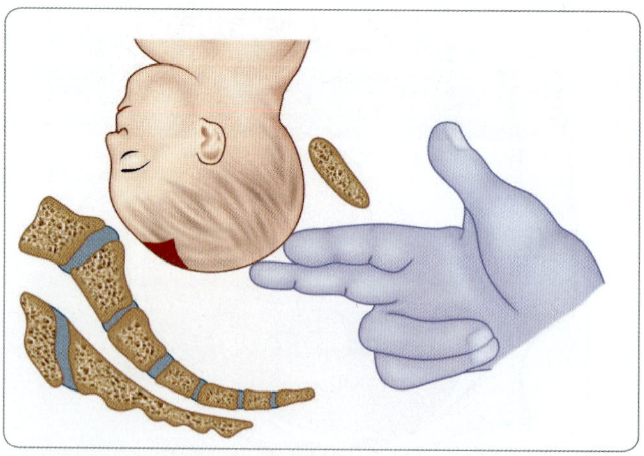

Fig. 4: Diagnosis of the position of the occiput. When the occiput is anterior it can be felt easily behind the symphysis pubis

At first the sagittal suture is identified. The sagittal suture is followed. On the one side it ends in the anterior fontanelle and on the other end is the posterior fontanelle. In occipitoposterior position the posterior fontanelle is located towards the sacro-iliac joint or may be directly towards the sacrum. The anterior fontanelle is easily palpable due to deflexion of the head (Fig. 5). From this fact the degree of deflexion can be assessed. Late in labor it might be difficult to identify the sutures owing to presence of caput succedaneum. In that case examination should be performed under general anesthesia. Examining fingers are introduced by the side of the head to feel the ear. The free border of the pina points towards the occiput.

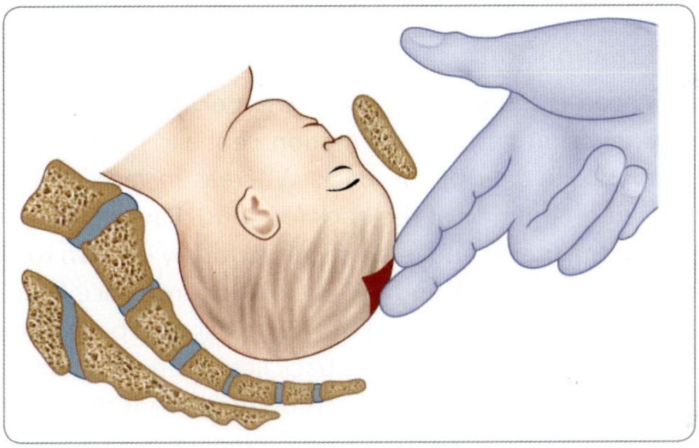

Fig. 5: Diagnosis of the position of the occiput. When the occiput is posterior the head is deflexed and the anterior fontanalle is felt anteriorly behind the symphysis pubis

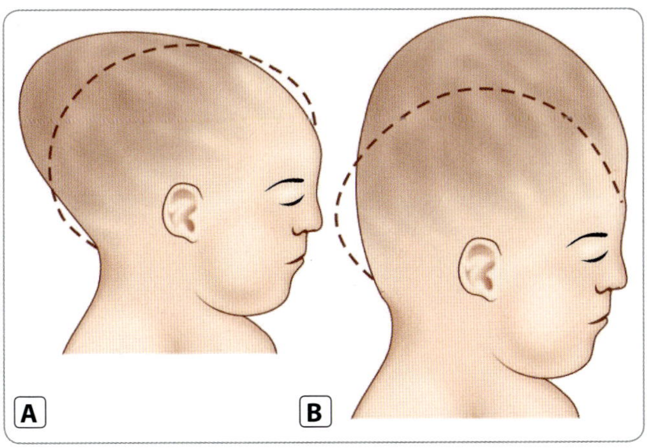

Figs 6A and B: Moulding of the fetal head in (A) Occipitoanterior and, (B) Occipitoposterior position. In occipitoposterior position there is increase in mento-vertical diameter

❒ FACE PRESENTATION

A face presentation is due to full extension of the fetal head on the neck. The occiput rests upon the upper back. Incidence of face presentation is about one in three hundred deliveries. Only rarely face presentation is found during pregnancy. It is usually diagnosed during labor.

Any one of the clinical factors described may be associated with face presentation. It is seen that in majority of cases face presentation is associated with fetal abnormality, particularly anencephaly. Congenital goiter preventing complete flexion of the head may cause face presentation. In some cases there may be increased spasm of the extensor group of muscles of the fetal neck promoting extension of the head. Contracted pelvis is another frequent accompaniment of face presentation.

Abdominal Examination

On pelvic grip head is found to lie above the pelvic brim with conspicuous cephalic prominence. In vertex presentation cephalic prominence (sinciput) is felt on the opposite side of the back. Whereas in face presentation the prominence is felt on the side of the back (occiput). Back of the fetus is felt in the upper part of the uterus and it is difficult to follow it down to the occiput. A gap is felt between the back and the occipital prominence (Fig. 8). This is a very characteristic sign of face presentation. But it should be remembered that this typical sign is found only when the back lies anteriorly. In case where the back is posterior or in other words in mento-anterior position the back is not felt anteriorly and similarly the occipital prominence is also not palpable. In these cases fetal limbs are felt more easily. When the back is anterior fetal heart sound is heard at a higher level than in vertex presentation and when the back is posterior fetal heart is heard directly over the chest.

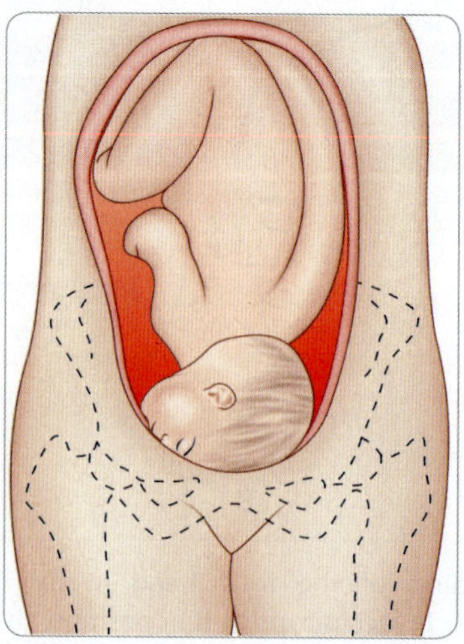

Fig. 7: Face presentation, mentoposterior position (right)

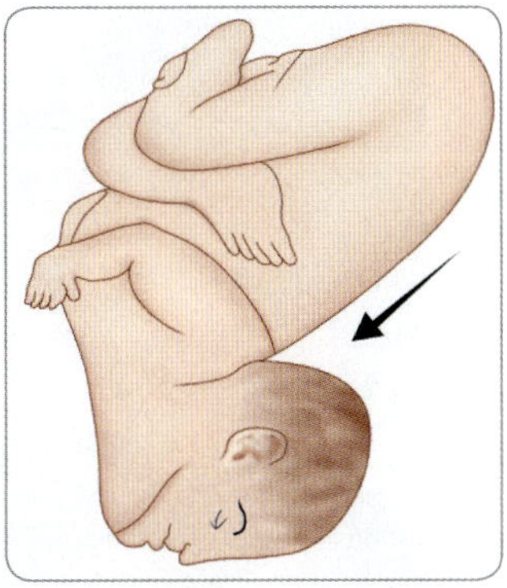

Fig. 8: Face presentation, note the deep groove (arrow) between the back and the occipital prominence

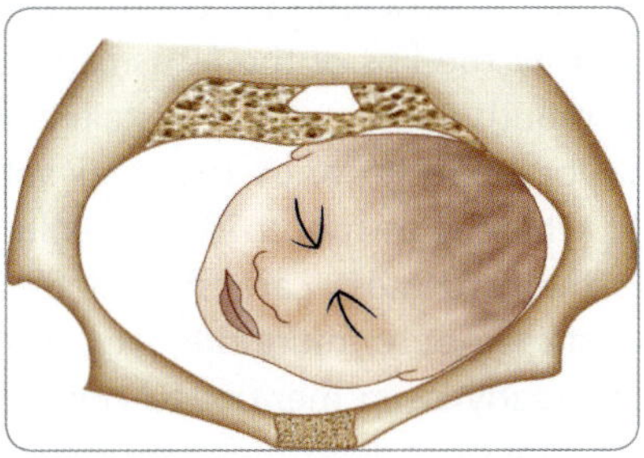

Fig. 9: Face presentation seen from below

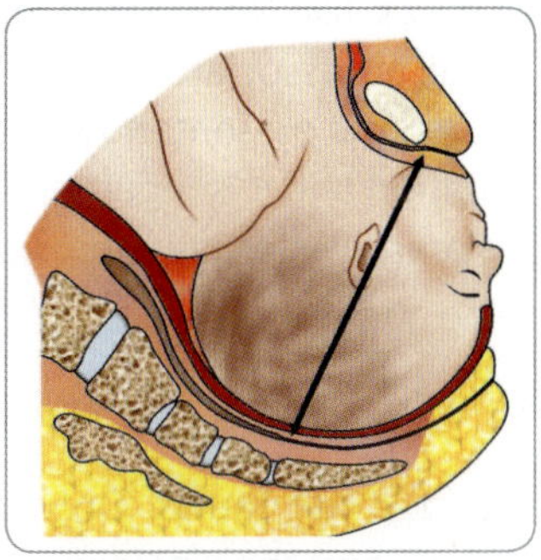

Fig. 10: Face presentation with submentovertical diameter

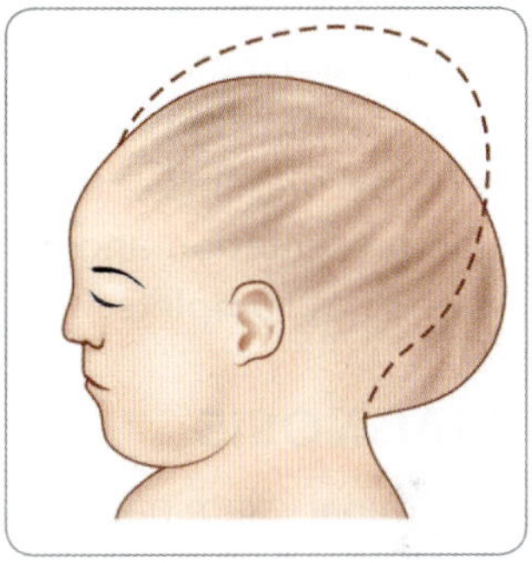

Fig. 11: Moulding of the fetal head in face presentation

Vaginal Examination

Vaginal examination done early in labor provides very little information as the presenting part lies high and it is difficult to outline. Only some soft part can be felt.

After few hours of labor membranes may be found in an elongated manner. Care should be taken not to rupture the membranes. Examination should be carried out during uterine relaxation. At this stage the frontal suture and the orbital ridges can be identified. If the frontal suture is followed after the orbital ridges the nose can be identified. Beyond this it is difficult to ascertain and if more attempt is made the membranes may rupture.

After rupture of membranes and when cervix is sufficiently dilated diagnosis is not difficult. Orbital ridges, mouth and chin can be felt. Special attention should be paid to the direction of the chin which indicates the position. The chin with two molar eminences makes a triangle. Inside the triangle is the mouth. Passing a finger gently inside the mouth the alveolar processes can be recognized by its firm margins. This is of particular importance when late in labor the face is obscured by edema. The sucking action of the lips of the fetus can be felt. But the mouth must not be mistaken to be the anal opening. In anus the anal sphincter is felt, whereas in mouth the alveolar margins are there. Utmost care should be taken at this stage not to injure the eyes, nose, etc. As has already been mentioned position of face presentation is determined by the direction of the chin.

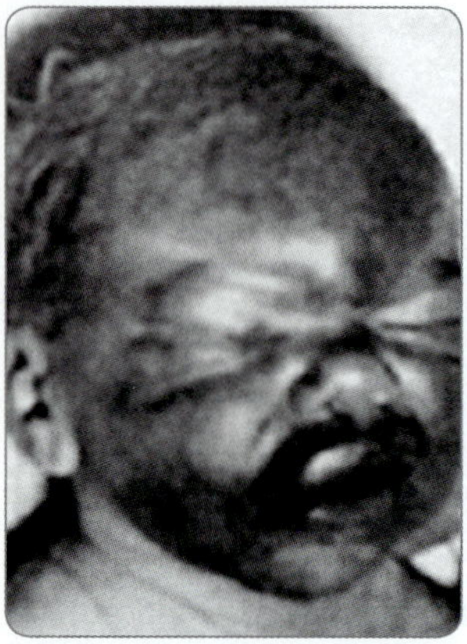

Fig. 12: Appearance of the face after delivery

❒ BROW PRESENTATION

In majority of persistent brow presentation factors like contracted pelvis, prematurity and multiparity with lax abdominal wall are associated with. When the head lies midway between flexion and extension the presentation is brow. The forehead presents at the brim. It is a rare condition and it is regarded as an unstable presentation and a sub-variety of face presentation as extension of the head is not complete.

❒ DIAGNOSIS

On abdominal examination adequate information is not found. Only thing is that the head remains high and both the occiput and the sinciput are felt almost at the same level.

Vaginal examination done early in labor is also not informative except the presence of an elongated bag of membranes which should arouse the suspicion of an abnormal presentation. Late in labor brow presentation can be

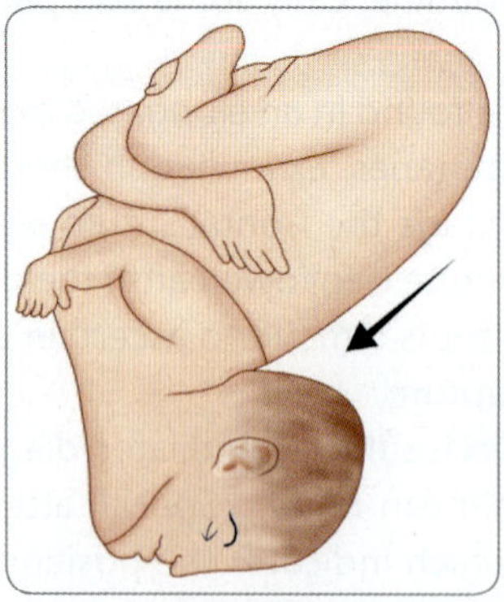

Fig. 13: Brow presentation. (note the deflexed attitude of the head)

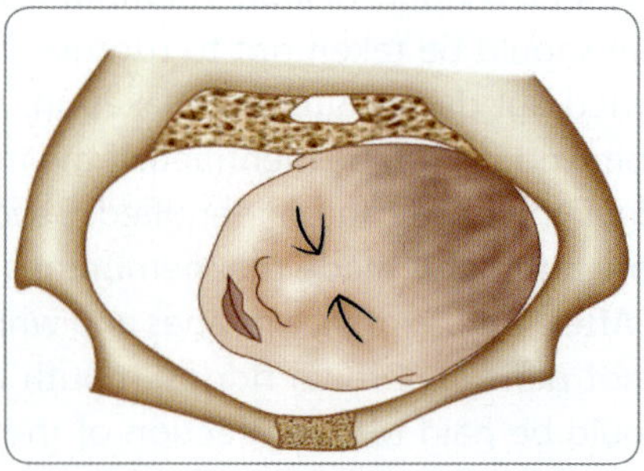

Fig. 14: Brow presentation (seen from below)

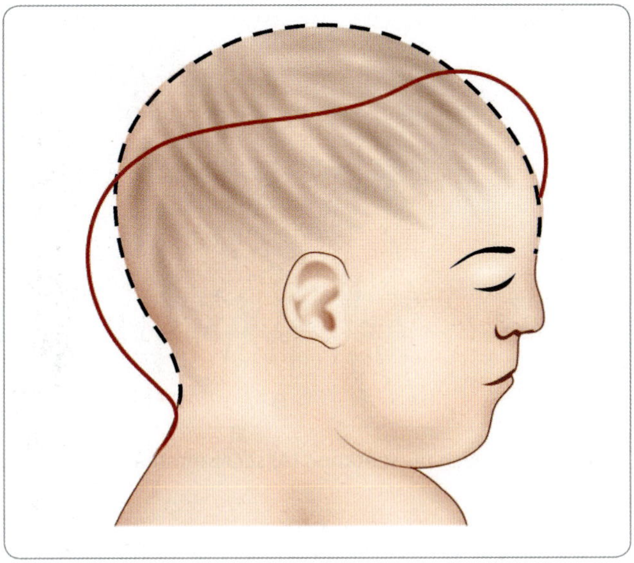

Fig. 15: Moulding of the fetal head in brow presentation (lengthening of the occipitofrontal diameter)

diagnosed by the presence of the anterior fontanelle on one side and orbital ridges on the other side of the presenting part.

❒ BREECH PRESENTATION

In breech presentation the lie is longitudinal with the podalic end at the brim of the pelvis and the cephalic end occupying the fundus of the uterus. Breech presentation occurs in about 3–4 percent of all labors. It is more frequent in preterm than in term deliveries. The incidence of breech presentation at 32 weeks of pregnancy is about 7 percent.

Types of Breech Presentation

When the podalic end of the fetus occupies the brim of the pelvis the presentation is breech.

The following are the types of breech presentation:

A. Complete breech or flexed breech presentation
B. Incomplete breech presentation.
   1. Breech with extended legs (Frank breech)
   2. Breech with extended thighs
      Knee flexed – knee presentation
      Knee extended – footling presentation.

In complete or flexed breech both knees and hips are flexed and feet are near the buttock. The presenting part consists of the buttock, the external genitalia and the feet. But in breech with extended legs the legs are flexed at

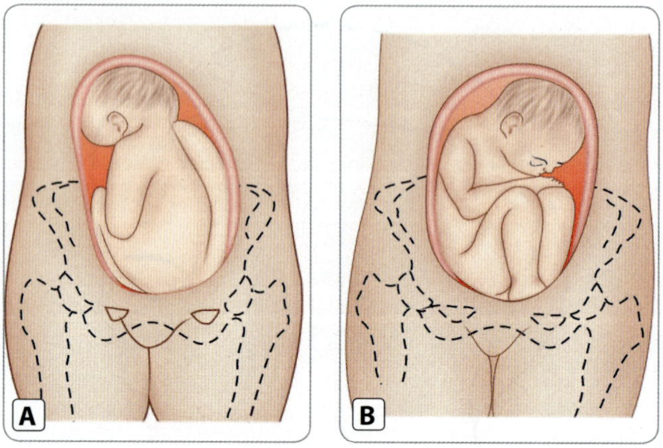

Figs 16A and B: Breech presentation (A) sacroanterior; (B) sacroposterior

the hips and extended at knees. The feet lie in the fundus of the uterus, at the side of the head. In this type the presenting part consists of the buttock and the external genitalia only. When the thighs are extended and knees flexed, the knees becomes the lower most and knee presentation results. Sometimes both hips and knees are partially extended and footling presentation results (Figs 17 and 18). Breech with extended legs is common and more frequent in primigravida than in multiparous women.

Causes

Some contributory conditions are found to be associated with breech presentation, but in many cases no such cause may be available. The contributory conditions of breech presentation are fetal malformation such as hydrocephalus. In this condition, the bigger head is well-accommodated in the wide fundal area of the uterus. In hydramnios owing to large volume of liquid amnii present the fetus can move easily and may present with any presentation. The next important associated condition is site of placentation. In case of placenta praevia due to the presence of the placenta in the lower uterine segment less space is available for the fetal head to remain there. In cornual attachment of the placenta head is well-accommodated in other corrnual end of the fundus and the bulky breech is pulled down into the lower uterine segment. Pelvic contraction is another condition which favors breech presentation. In Miillerian abnormality such as bicornuate uterus, uterine diadelphus breech presentation is found more frequently. Genetic disorders that alter the fetal muscular tone and mobility also favors breech presentation.

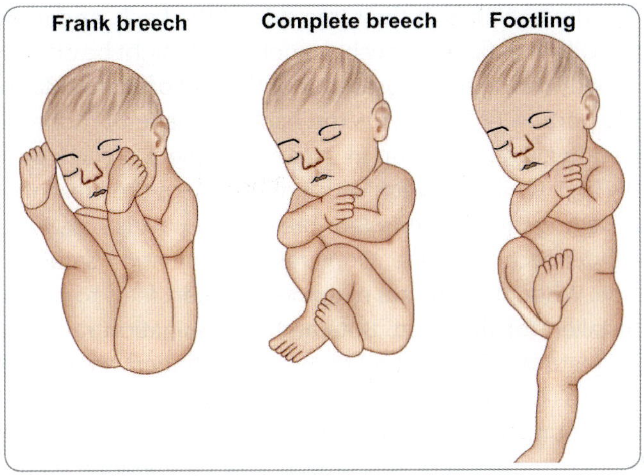

Fig. 17: Different breech presentation

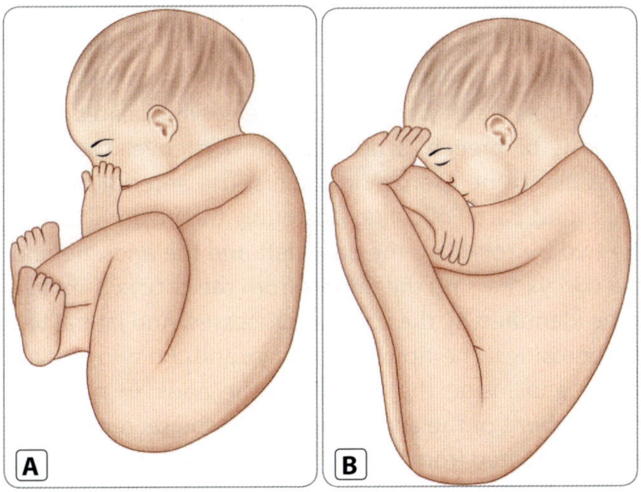

Figs 18A and B: Breech presentation (A) with flexed leg, (B) with extended leg

❒ DIAGNOSIS

One important feature in history of the woman with breech presentation is that the patient often complains of pain over one or the other hypochondrium, owing to the presence of the head of the fetus at that region.

Abdominal Examination

In fundal grip the head can be recognized by its characteristic features. It is hard, smooth, round mass. In case of complete breech, the head lies to the side of the midline opposite to the side of the back. Whereas in breech with extended legs the head lies to the same side of the back. And in this case the head is not mobile as in flexed breech. Sometimes it might be difficult to outline the head properly owing to the presence of the feet on both sides of the head. In the middle portion of the uterus the back can be felt on one side and the limbs on the other. On pelvic grip in case of complete breech, the presenting part is usually high while in breech with extended legs the presenting part may be found to be engaged. In complete breech the part is soft, irregular, bulky and less well-defined in outline. On careful examination small parts can be felt to the side. When the legs are extended the part feels to be firm and may easily be mistaken for the head. But careful examination reveals absence of characteristic features of the head and when the fingers are pushed down no resistance is felt as it would be in vertex presentation.

Fetal heart sound is usually heard at or slightly above the level of the umbilicus. With extended legs the breech may be engaged early and so the level at which fetal heart sound is best heard may be lower.

Vaginal Examination

Early in labor in complete breech the presenting part lies high at the brim. Through the insufficiently dilated cervix elongated bag of membranes is found. The buttock is felt as a soft part only. As the cervix dialates and membranes rupture diagnosis of breech is not difficult. Moreover the presenting part is easily accessible to the examining fingers. The anterior buttock is felt as a soft, smooth, round part. Following posterioly the posterior buttock is felt. In between the two buttocks are the anal cleft and the anus. Behind the anus is the tip of the coccyx. Passing the fingers from the coccyx the sacrum is found. Sacrum can be identified by the spinous processes. And lateral to the anus are two ischial tuberosities. The tip of the coccyx and the two ischial tuberosities form a triangle and inside the triangle is the anus. In male baby external genitalia is felt in front of the anus. Opposite to the sacrum the feet are felt. A foot can be differentiated from hand by the presence of the heel and the great toe which cannot be abducted.

In breech with extended legs other findings are the same as in complete breech except the absence of feet with buttock. In knee and footling presentations recognition of the feet is all that is necessary. Another characteristic feature is the passage of meconium which can be seen in vulva late in labor. In breech presentation sacrum is the denominator. For determination of position the direction of the sacrum is important to note.

❒ SHOULDER PRESENTATION (TRANSVERSE LIE)

In shoulder presentation the long axis of the fetus lies transversely or obliquely. This presentation occurs in about 2.4 percent of all labors.

The causes of malpresentation such as contracted pelvis, preterm labor, polyhydramnios, placenta previa, Miillerian abnormality of the uterus, lax anterior abdominal wall, etc. are frequently found with shoulder presentation.

❐ DIAGNOSIS

During Pregnancy

During later weeks of pregnancy diagnosis of transverse or oblique lie is not difficult by abdominal examination. If systematic examination is carried out the following features will be noted. The shape of the uterus is not a typically eliptical one as in longitudinal lie. With transverse lie the uterus is asymmetrical, irregular and more wider than in longitudinal lie. Fundus remains at a lower level for corresponding period of gestation. On fundal grip the fundus is found to be empty. Head is felt in one iliac fossa and the breech occupies the opposite one but at a higher level (Fig. 19). Usually the back is anterior. If the back is posterior limbs can be felt anteriorly. On pelvic grip the lower pole of the uterus is found empty. Fetal heart sound is heard over the back. Vaginal examination at this stage is of no help in diagnosis.

During Labor

Early in labor before rupture of membranes abdominal findings are same as in pregnancy. Vaginal examination reveals an elongated bag of membranes in which small fetal arm may be felt. After rupture of membranes an arm may prolapse and very often accompanies a loop of umbilical cord.

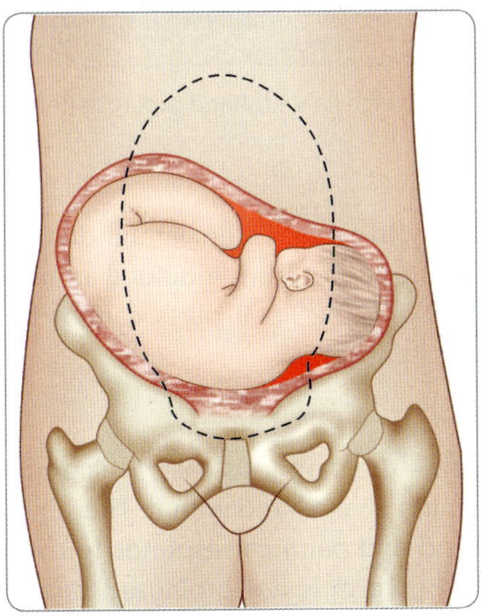

Fig. 19: Transverse lie (note the shape of the uterus; dotted line shows the normal shape)

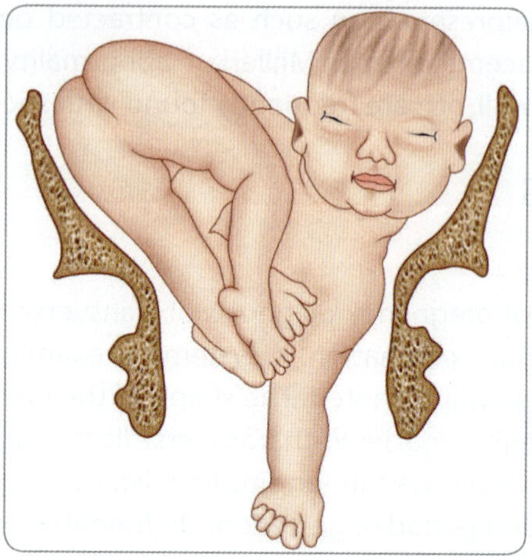

Fig. 20: Transverse lie with hand prolapse

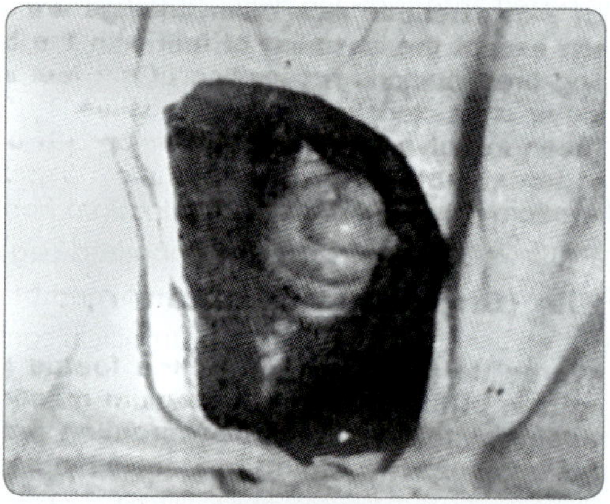

Fig. 21: Transverse lie with hand prolapse (fetus is living)

Late in Labor

Membranes rupture early in labor. Liquor amnii drains out with or without prolapse of an arm. The uterus becomes moulded around the fetus and makes abdominal examination difficult. Fetal parts cannot be identified properly. Fetal heart sound is almost absent.

Vaginal Examination

Prolapse of an arm makes the diagnosis easy. Which hand has prolapsed can be made out by imagining shake hand with it. Thumb of the supinated hand directs towards the head and palm corresponds to the ventral aspect of the fetus. In those cases when arm is not prolapsed careful examination of the presenting part is needed. Pushing the examining fingers inside the vagina a soft mass is felt. Beneath the soft tissue ribs can be felt which run parallel

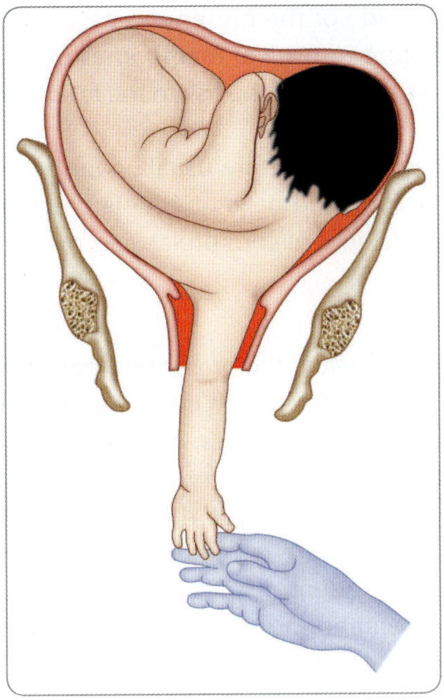

Fig. 22: Transverse lie with hand prolapse, diagnosis of position by "Shake hand" method

to each other with intercostal space in between. When the ribs are followed they end in the vertebral spines. On further exploration tip of the scapula is felt which is freely mobile and projects from the surface of the back. When fingers are passed across the ribs on either side apex of the axila is found on one side. Axillary pit points towards the head. Before taking out the fingers accessibility of neck should be assessed.

❒ COMPOUND PRESENTATION

Sometimes an arm may descend along with the head. The hand may be below the head or at the side. Very rarely a foot also comes down. This is called compound presentation or complex presentation. The condition is usually seen with contracted pelvis and with premature baby. In an average size pelvis with an average size baby there will be delay in labor. Diagnosis is made by vaginal examination when a hand is found with the head.

Cord Presentation and Cord Prolapse

Descent of the umbilical cord below the presenting part is a grave condition for the fetus. The cord may come down before or after rapture of membrane. When descent occurs before rupture of membranes it is called cord presentation and descent after rupture of membranes is called cord prolapse. Sometimes the cord may remain at the side of the presenting part and is not actually below the presenting part. Before rupture of membranes pressure of the presenting part over the cord is less and hence the risk to the fetus is also less, but warrants urgent intervention.

Cord presentation and prolapse are usually found in breech and shoulder presentations or with contracted pelvis, multiple pregnancy and hydramnios. In premature baby the incident of cord prolapse is more.

❒ DIAGNOSIS

Presence of umbilical cord below the presenting part can be easily diagnosed by its pulsation. But in a dead fetus with intact membranes recognition might be difficult. After rupture of membranes, of course, there is no difficulty. The condition is diagnosed only by vaginal examination, and the fetus is at great risk after rupture of membranes. So it should be a routine practice to do vaginal examination after rupture of membranes, particularly with abnormal presentation or with high presenting part at the time of rupture.

Except in vertex presentation in all other presentations soft tissue is there in the presenting part. Late in labor it is difficult to recognize the parts easily owing to swelling and edema. The diagnostic landmarks of these presentations should be kept in mind and searched for. Moreover, a systematic abdominal examination should always preced a vaginal examination.

In breech presentation with extended legs and typical characteristics of the head may not be found owing to the presence of the legs beside the head and the breech may be felt like a head or the breech may be deep into the pelvis. In that case the size of the presenting part should be assessed comparing with the size of the baby.

On vaginal examination presence of the anus with anal sphincter and external genitalis in male baby confirms the diagnosis. In face presentation inside the mouth there is the alveolar margin with firm feeling and sometimes sucking action of the lips are helpful for diagnosis. Presence of the ribs and the tip of the scapula confirms shoulder presentation without hand prolapse. If needed radiological examination or ultrasonography is helpful to confirm the diagnosis of abnormal presentation.

chapter 16 Multiple Pregnancy

Multiple pregnancy is of high risk category because of several complications associated with it. Perinatal mortality and morbidity are very high. Twin pregnancy is the commonest variety of multiple pregnancy. Twins are either **monozygotic** or **dizygotic**. Monozygotic twin results from splitting of a single fertilized ovum and develops into two distinct individuals. Such individuals are genetically identical and of similar sex. Dizygotic twins result from fertilization of two different ovum by different spermatozoa. The individuals are genetically different and the sex may vary.

❒ INCIDENCE

Incidence of monozygotic twin appears to be relatively constant throughout the world at the rate of approximately 4 per 1000 births. The rate is independent of maternal age, parity, race or heredity. The incidence of dizygotic twin is influenced by maternal age, parity and ethnicity. Use of artificial reproductive technology has largely increased the incidence of multiple pregnancy. Use of gonadotropin and clomiphene citrate is associated with increase in the number of multiple pregnancy. In vitro fertilization and embryo transfer has further increased the incidence.

❒ PLACENTATION

In a singleton pregnancy the fetus develops inside a sac consisting of two membranes – a chorion outside and an amnion inside. Placenta develops in chorion. In dizygotic twin two individuals develop inside their own sacs consisting of both the chorion and amnion. Placenta is also two in number. If implantation takes place side by side, intimate fusion of the two placentas may occur, usually having no vascular connection. These placentas are always diamnionic and dichorionic.

The type of placenta that develops in monozygotic twin pregnancy is determined by the timing of splitting of the fertilized ovum. If splitting occurs within the first 3 days after fertilization, before formation of inner cell mass, i.e. before setting aside the cells which will form the chorion, two embryos, two chorions and two amnions will develop. There will be a diamnionic dichorionic monozygotic twins.

If splitting occurs between fourth and eighth day, after inner cell mass is formed, embryos will develop within a single chorion with two separate amnions. Thus a diamnionic monochorionic monozygotic twin will develop. Between 8th and 13th day amnion has already developed and splitting at that time will result in a monoamnionic monochorionic monozygotic twin. Embryonic splitting will result in conjoined twin within a single amnion and single chorion, as splitting at this time is incomplete.

❐ COMPLICATIONS

Multiple pregnancy is an abnormal pregnancy associated with increased maternal and perinatal complications.

Common problems of pregnancy are increased. There may be severe vomiting in early pregnancy. Similarly tiredness, breathlessness in mid-pregnancy is increased. There may be early onset pedal edema, varicose vein and piles, etc.

The frequency of pre-eclampsia and eclampsia is more in multiple pregnancy. She may suffer from anaemia which may be iron deficiency anemia or megaloblastic anemia from folate deficiency. Placenta in multiple pregnancy is large in size or there may be two separate placenta. There is more chance that the placenta encroaches upon the lower uterine segment resulting in placenta previa. Malpresentation is another common feature of multiple pregnancy.

Preterm labor is the single most common cause of increased perinatal mortality in multiple pregnancy. Labor is usually prolonged in multiple pregnancy and often with early rupture of membranes. There is increased risk of sepsis if labor is unduly prolonged. As the uterus is overdistended and uterine inertia is common, there is a real danger of developing postpartum hemorrhage. After delivery of the first baby there is great risk of accidental hemorrhage.

Perinatal mortality and morbidity in multiple pregnancy is approximately three times greater than in singleton pregnancy. Perinatal mortality in twin due to pre-maturity is about six times higher than in singleton delivery. Intrauterine growth restriction is another major factor for increased death rate. Both intrauterine death and early neonatal death are more common in monozygotic twin. Again in monozygotic twin presence of inter-twin vascular shunt increases the risk. Twins also have increased incidence of congenital anomaly. Twins are more likely to have neurological impairment and lower IQ. Besides, incidence of cerebral palsy is quite high among the twins than among the singleton babies.

❐ PREDISPOSING FACTORS

It is observed that few factors predispose to the occurrence of twin pregnancy. In certain ethnic groups twins are more common. It is found that in some race of Nigeria incidence of twin pregnancy is very high whereas in Japan the incidence is low. As a whole the incidence of dizygotic twin is less among the Asian population.

Twining is more common among those women who themselves were dizygotic twin. It is observed that in determining twining genotype of the mother is important. Maternal age and parity have some positive effect on twining. Higher the age and parity of the woman, higher is the chance of having multiple pregnancy. In recent years, use of artificial reproductive technology has greatly increased the incidence of multiple births. Drugs used for ovulation induction and in vitro fertilization and embryo transfer have contributed to the incidence of multiple pregnancy and have evolved techniques like selective reduction of fetus and/or selective termination of defective fetus, etc.

❒ DIAGNOSIS

Before routine use of ultrasonography in obstetrics most of the twins were diagnosed during labor only. The possibility of twin pregnancy should be considered if the early pregnancy discomforts like vomiting, tiredness are exaggerated. In such situation if the mother herself was a twin or if there is history of previous twin pregnancy the obstetrician should remember the possibility of twin pregnancy. In later weeks of pregnancy, the woman experiences undue heavyness of lower abdomen and even walking may be difficult, turning on bed from one side to another becomes troublesome. She may complain of excessive fetal movement.

On physical examination early pedal edema in a multiparous woman should arouse the suspicion of multiple pregnancy. She is more prone to develop symptoms of pre-eclampsia, anemia and varicose vein on legs.

On abdominal examination size of the uterus is more than the period of gestation. Multiple fetal parts are felt. In presence of hydramnios or in obese women it may be difficult to palpate the fetal parts. In thin women two fetal heads and too many fetal parts may be felt to confirm the diagnosis of twin pregnancy. Another diagnostic feature of twin pregnancy is detection of two fetal heart sounds, their points of maximal intensity being at different positions with faded or no sound area in between. Fetal heart sound should be counted by two observers over at least one minute and the difference in rate should be at least 10 beats per minute.

When diagnosis of twin pregnancy is made only during delivery, the uterus remains at a higher level after birth of the first baby. On palpation of the abdomen the second fetus can be felt and on vaginal examination another bag of membrane is felt with the presenting part of the fetus.

❒ ULTRASONOGRAPHY

With ultrasonography multiple pregnancy can be diagnosed early in pregnancy. Separate gestation sac can be identified by about 6 weeks of gestation (Fig. 1).

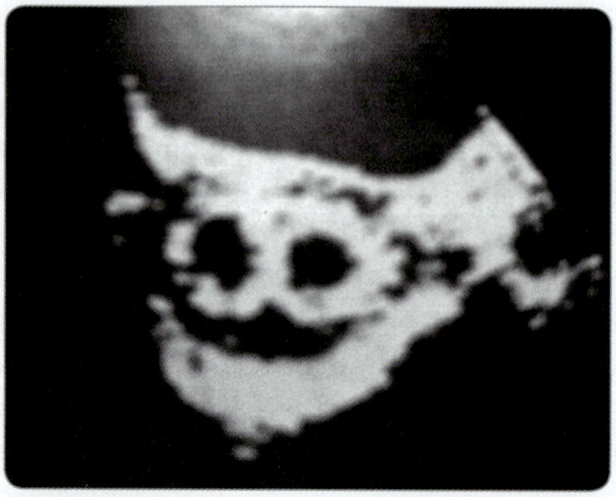

Fig. 1: Ultrasonography of twin pregnancy showing two sacs of 5 weeks' pregnancy

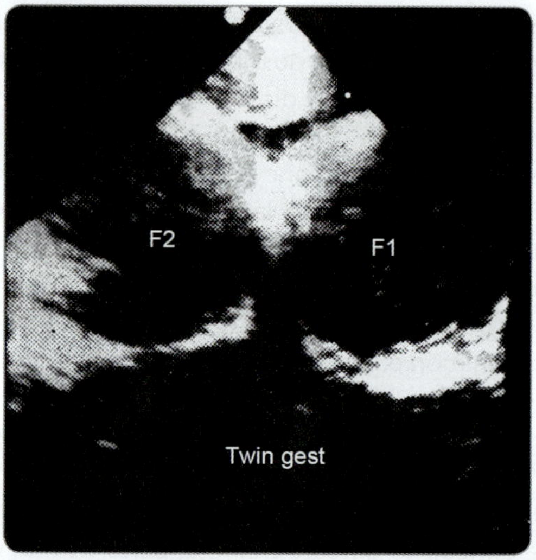

Fig. 2: Ultrasonography of twin pregnancy

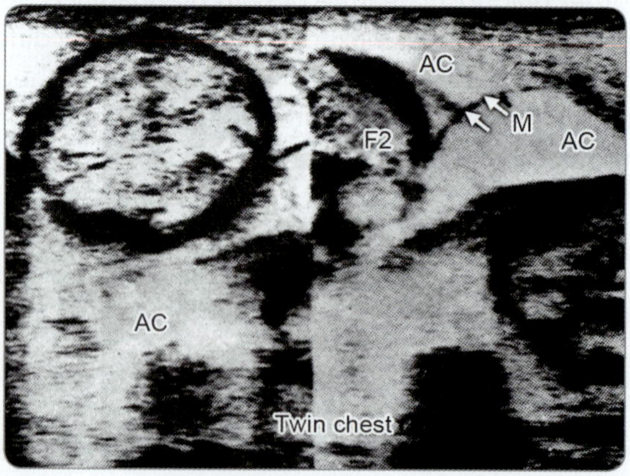

Fig. 3: Ultrasonography of twin pregnancy – note the amniotic membrane between two sacs

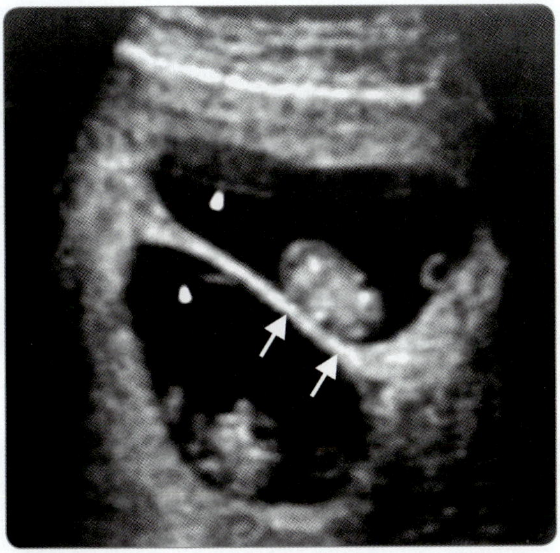

Fig. 4: Ultrasonography of twin pregnancy showing inter-twin membrane

Embryos in two sacs can be visualized by transabdominal ultrasonography by 7 weeks and individual heart beats after 7 weeks of pregnancy. By transvaginal sonography fetal heart can be identified by 6 weeks of pregnancy and intracranial landmarks can be identified by 10–12 weeks which are visualized by 13–14 weeks by transabdominal scanning. Fetal yolk sac should be identified in each sac.

Sometimes one sac may remain anembryonic and may lead to vanishing twin. There may be spontaneous stoppage of heart beat in one sac followed by resorption of the embryo and the sac. Incidence of IUGR and fetal death are higher in monochorionic twins than in dichorionic twins. Twin-to-twin transfusion occurs only in monochorionic twins. Chorionicity and amnionicity can be determined by careful ultrasonographic examination. Pregnancy is dichorionic if two separate placentas with different sex of the fetuses are seen. When single placenta is seen with same sex of the fetus the intervening membrane is examined carefully particularly for its thickness and number of layers visualized. In dichorionic diamnionic twin the intervening membrane appears thick.

Ideally the initial scan is advised around 10–14 weeks of gestation. Subsequently it should be repeated periodically to detect congenital abnormality and to assess fetal growth.

❐ EXAMINATION OF PLACENTA

After the expulsion of the placentas the intervening membrane should be examined. If it consists only two membranes (amnion) without intervening

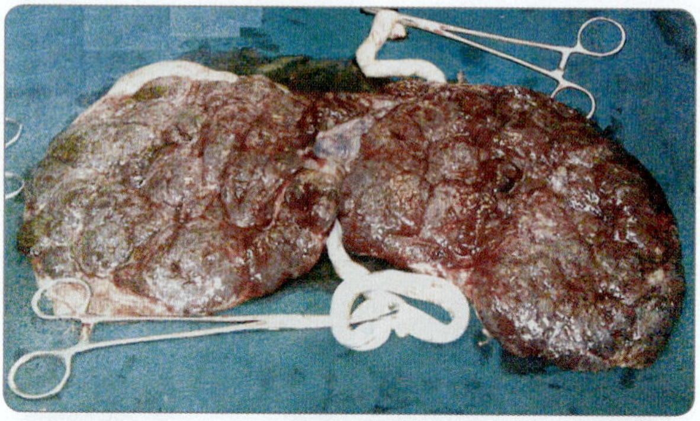

Fig. 5: Placenta of binovular twin with fused margin (maternal surface)

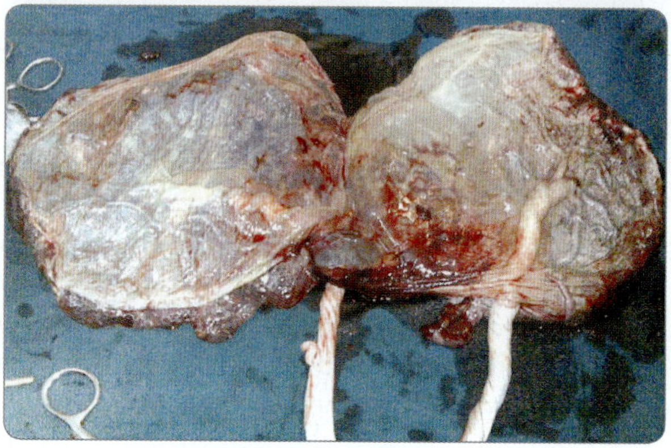

Fig. 6: Placenta of binovular twin with fused margin (fetal surface)

chorion the infants are monozygotic. If adjacent amnions are separated by chorion the fetuses may be dizygotic or monozygotic. If infants are of different sex they are dizygotic. But in case of same sex blood group examination is needed to ascertain the zygocity of the infants.

chapter

17 Intrauterine Growth Restrictions

Some fetuses fail to achieve the normal growth potential. In intrauterine growth restriction the fetus fails to achieve the expected weight for a given period of gestation. The term intrauterine growth restriction (IUGR) is preferred to intrauterine growth retardation. A small for gestational age baby (SGA) is one whose birth weight is below the 10th percentile for the corresponding gestational age and a low birth weight (LBW) baby is one whose birth weight is less than 2500 g at term. A SGA baby may not be growth restricted. These terms are not synonymous and there is overlapping.

The perinatal mortality rate for IUGR babies are 6–10 times higher than that for normally-grown babies. IUGR is associated with a large number of stillbirths.

❒ ETIOLOGY

There is a wide range of conditions fetal, maternal and environmental that are associated with intrauterine growth restriction. Still in many cases no definite associated condition can be detected and the etiology may remain obscure.

Maternal Causes

A constitutionally small woman, otherwise healthy may deliver a small baby without any other problem. This group of baby needs no treatment.

Maternal Disease

Certain maternal diseases such as pre-eclampsia; essential hypertension, chronic renal disease leads to intrauterine growth restriction due to utero-placental insufficiency. Women suffering from cyanotic heart disease or chronic pulmonary disease cause chronic hypoxia and eventually lead to growth restriction of the fetus.

Smoking

Smoking is an important cause of intrauterine growth restrictions. Male fetuses are more commonly affected than the female. It may be due to increased concentration of carboxy hemoglobin in fetus of smoking mothers than in non-smoking mothers. Again there may be adverse effect on utero-placental circulation.

Alcohol

Chronic consumption of moderate to heavy amount of alcohol by the mother during pregnancy results in growth restriction of the fetus.

Drugs

Use of drugs such as cocaine and heroin is associated with impairment of fetal growth and eventually intrauterine growth restriction.

Infection

Malaria is a common cause of growth restriction. Herpes, rubella, cytomegalovirus, toxoplasmosis and syphilis can lead to smallness of fetus.

Genetic Causes

Chromosomal abnormalities and congenital malformation are found to be associated with intrauterine growth impairment. Growth is impaired early in pregnancy and growth restriction is of symmetric type.

Multiple Pregnancy

Where two or more fetuses are present, growth is likely to be restricted leading to delivery of small babies.

Maternal Nutrition

Maternal nutritional support is an important factor for adequate fetal growth. Deficiency of adequate nutritional supply to the mother may result in growth restriction in third trimester of pregnancy.

Placental Cause

Placenta is the organ through which the fetus gets nutrition and oxygen from the mother. Uteroplacental insufficiency from any cause leads to growth restriction. Many conditions mentioned above lead to placental insufficiency, resulting in growth-restricted fetuses. In a placenta of smaller size maternal supply to the fetus is reduced, thereby producing a small fetus. Similarly abnormalities of the placenta also may lead to growth restriction. Conditions like circumvallate placenta, partial separation of placenta, infarction and hemangioma may cause IUGR. Abnormal localization of placenta like placenta previa is associated with an increased risk to IUGR.

❒ DIAGNOSIS

History: Careful history taking may reveal presence of predisposing factors of the above mentioned medical conditions which may lead to IUGR babies. The attending doctor should be concerned about the risk of the fetus in presence of such history.

Clinical examination to assess the size of the uterus is important to suspect IUGR. If the increase in size of uterus does not correlates with the period of gestation fetal growth restriction is suspected. A better parameter to assess the growth of the uterus is measurement of symphysis fundal height. In western countries the average symphysis fundal height was within one centimeter of gestational age in weeks. If the fundal height is 4 cm or more less than the corresponding gestational age growth restriction should be suspected.

❒ ULTRASONOGRAPHY

Clinical Examination

If intrauterine growth restriction is suspected ultrasonographic examination is needed to confirm the diagnosis. On ultrasonographic examination, fetal weight is estimated from different measurements of the fetal body. Fetal growth being a dynamic process needs serial evaluation to arrive at a diagnosis. Fetal biometry includes measurement of biparietal diameter (BPD), abdominal circumference (AC), and head circumference, femur length, etc. In suspected cases if the estimated fetal weight falls below 10th percentile for the corresponding gestational age serial evaluation is to be done, at least at a gap of 3 weeks.

In case of asymmetrical IUGR head circumference is larger than the abdominal circumference. In symmetrical IUGR both head circumference and abdominal circumference are reduced. A single ultrasonographic screening of the fetus and the gestation as a whole in early weeks of pregnancy is very valuable for future estimation of fetal age and for planning the mode of delivery.

Decreased amniotic fluid volume or oligohydramnios is often associated with intrauterine growth restriction.

chapter

18 Intrauterine Fetal Death

The fetus may die in its intrauterine life before onset of labor. Death is usually followed by spontaneous expulsion of the fetus. Very rarely expulsion may be delayed. It is estimated that maximum number of fetal death occurs before 32 weeks of gestation and women above 35 years of age are at greater risk for intrauterine fetal death than women under 30 years.

❐ CAUSES

Complications of Pregnancy

Few complications of pregnancy when remain untreated or inadequately treated may lead to death of the fetus. Pregnancy induced hypertension is a common condition associated with intrauterine fetal death. Severe pre-eclampsia and eclampsia are major causes of fetal death. Another effect of pre-eclampsia on the fetus is intrauterine growth restriction (IUGR). Severe pre-eclampsia in association with IUGR increases the risk of fetal death by many folds. The causes of fetal death here is chronic asphyxia of the fetus. Similarly essential hypertension and chronic nephritis are likely to cause fetal demise unless adequately treated. Pregnancy induced hypertension is a frequent cause of accidental hemorrhage which is again a major contributor to intrauterine fetal death. Accidental hemorrhage leads to separation of a portion of placenta causing acute fetal asphyxia and death.

The incidence of gestational diabetes is increasing. When adequately taken care of and a normoglycemic state is maintained throughout pregnancy intrauterine fetal death is rare. But inadequately treated cases may remain hyperglycemic and causes macrosomia, hydramnios, pre-eclampsia and there may even be vascular disease leading to fetal death. In diabetes mellitus fetal death is more common around 35–36 weeks of gestation.

Severe anemia is another important cause of intrauterine death. Rh-isoimmunization rarely may lead to hydrops fetalis and eventually fetal death.

Fetal malformations which are not compatible with life may cause intrauterine fetal death.

Post-maturity or post-dated pregnancy may cause intrauterine death without much prior warning. IUGR and placental insufficiency from any cause lead to fetal death. Most of the deaths from IUGR occur during later weeks of pregnancy.

Intrauterine infection is an important cause of fetal death in utero. Also a special group of organisms infect the placenta and the fetus. Infections caused by this group of organisms are known as `TORCH' infections. Here T is for toxoplasmosis,'O is for other infections like syphilis, hepatitis B and C, varicella, parvovirus B19, HIV, etc. R is for rubella infection, C is for cytomegalovirus and H is for herpes simplex infections. Depending on the time of infection during the gestational period there may be abortion, premature labor or even intrauterine fetal death.

Transmission of toxoplasma from the infected mother to the fetus can cause intrauterine death. Fetus is effected only when the mother suffers from acute toxoplasmosis. Rubella infection is usually acquired during the first 20 weeks of gestation and causes fetal damage. Regarding cytomegalovirus infection it is suggested that the infection is unlikely to cause spontaneous abortion or fetal death. In severe infection of herpes simplex virus fetal death may occur.

In many cases the exact cause of fetal death is not known. In about 20 percent of cases the etiology remains obscure.

❐ DIAGNOSIS

Signs and symptoms of intrauterine fetal death are different according to the period of gestation when death occurs. Fetal death may occur in early weeks of gestation or during mid-pregnancy or late in pregnancy and the signs and symptoms varies accordingly.

When fetal death occurs in early weeks of pregnancy, the uterus usually expels it in the form of abortion. Sometimes the uterus fails to expel it and the dead products of conception remain inside the uterus. Symptoms of pregnancy gradually diminishes and ultimately disappears. Breast tenderness and tenseness reduces.

There may be brown or dirty discharge per vagina.

On vaginal examination the size of the uterus is felt to the smaller than the period of gestation and examining fingers may be smeared with dirty discharge. Urine for pregnancy test may remain positive for sometime. The diagnosis may be confirmed by ultrasonographic examination. On ultrasonography the embryo may be absent or if present is without cardiac activity. Sac is deformed and there may be evidence of subchorionic bleed. If diagnosis is still in doubt repeat examination after about 7–10 days confirms the diagnosis.

If fetal death occurs in early second trimester symptoms and signs will be same as in first trimester and ultrasonographic examination can confirm the diagnosis.

In fetal death during the second trimester the woman will complain of absence of fetal movement. But many women fail to notice fetal activity for quite sometime. On examination there is cessation of gradual growth of the uterus which is characteristic of normal pregnancy. In some cases even the size of the uterus is found to be less than the period of gestation. Fetal movement is not felt and fetal heart sound is not audible. Sometimes even if the fetus is alive it is very difficult to ascertain fetal heart sound in cases of hydramnios or in obese women where anterior abdominal wall is very thick.

Diagnosis can be confirmed by radiology or by ultrasonography.

❒ RADIOLOGICAL SIGNS OF FETAL DEATH

The important radiological signs of fetal death are:

Marked overlapping of the skull bones. This is known as spalding sign. This is a characteristic sign of intrauterine fetal death. This is caused by liquifaction of brain matter. It takes several days to develop this sign. Similar type of overlapping, though to a lesser degree, may be seen in a living baby in labor. This is due to moulding of the fetal head.

Exaggerated curvature of the fetal spine is another important sign. This sign also needs several days to appear.

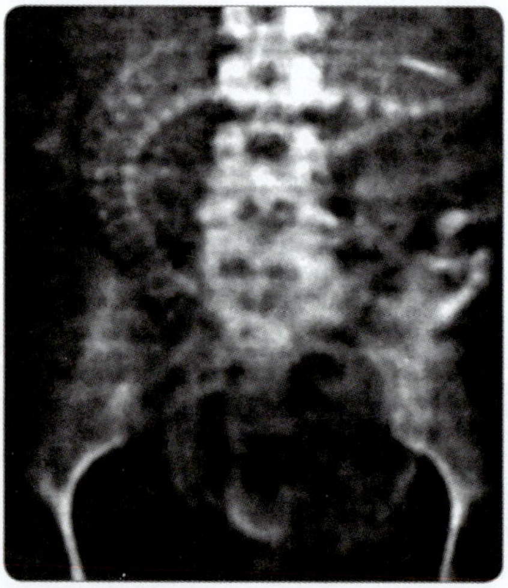

Fig. 1: Skiagram showing intrauterine fetal death (Note the spalding sign and hyperflexion of fetal spine)

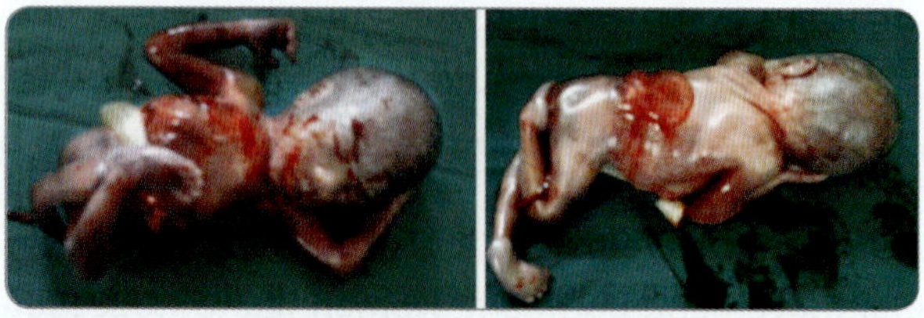

Fig. 2: Intrauterine death at 30 weeks of pregnancy. Fetus showing hydrocephalus and meningocele

Presence of gas shadow in big vessels is a reliable sign of fetal death but it is not commonly seen.

❐ ULTRASONOGRAPHIC SIGNS

In intrauterine death of the fetus fetal activity is found to be absent, when examined for 2–3 minutes. If needed, examination should be carried out by two examiners. Absence of cardiac activity is a sure sign of fetal demise.

chapter 19

Identification of High Risk Pregnancy

A pregnancy is said to be a high-risk one where the pregnancy outcome is likely to be undesirable. In developed countries maternal mortality is not more than the mortality among the general population. Naturally in those countries attention of the obstetricians has been focused on well-being of the unborn child. But the situation is not similar in the third world countries, where maternal mortality is still very high. In these countries obstetricians are equally concerned about the well-being of the mother also.

Some conditions, which might be social, economical or medical are known to influence the course and outcome of pregnancy and the ultimate result might not be favorable. These conditions are risk factors and should be identified at the time of first booking. Management of pregnancy and labor depends to a great extent on these risk factors.

To identify the risk factors a thorough history is essential. Detail history taking is the first step to highlight the possible factors. The next step is systematic physical examination of the patient. Any factor identified should be noted clearly and separately in the history sheet.

❒ THE RISK FACTORS AND THEIR POSSIBLE EFFECTS

Age

Pregnant woman below 18 years of age is known as young primigravida. In many cases these are unplanned pregnancy and the young lady is more prone to develop pre-eclampsia and eclampsia. On the other hand above 38 years of age a pregnant woman may have some problems. With advancing age medical disorders such as diabetes mellitus, hypertension, cardiac problems may aggravate and may adversely influence the course and outcome of the pregnancy. Moreover, in an elderly woman incidence of Down's syndrome of the fetus is more.

Parity

If a woman becomes pregnant for the first time after 35 years of age, she is known as elderly primigravida. She may have some problems as has been mentioned. Moreover, she is a good candidate to develop pregnancy induced hypertension and hence fetoplacental dysfunction. How a primigravida behaves during labor is not known. Her bony pelvis is not verified and hence primigravidity itself is considered as a risk factor.

If a woman delivers 5 or more than 5 times after 20 weeks of gestation she is known as grand multipara. A grand multipara is likely to develop anemia, abortion, antepartum and postpartum hemorrhage besides feto-placental dysfunctions.

Socio-economic Conditions

Pregnancy complications such as anemia, malnutrition and eclampsia are very common among the women from low socio-economic strata. Poverty, lack of education, ignorance and inadequate communication facilities from rural areas are main contributing factors for high maternal and perinatal mortality in these women.

Marital Status

Very often a young primigravida is not married and some other pregnant women may be divorcee or widow. In these cases the pregnancy is usually neglected and antenatal care is irregular or may not be at all. The woman is likely to be under severe mental stress.

Menstrual History

A good number of pregnant women are unaware of their last menstrual period and obstetrician is uncertain of the gestational age. Similar situation may arise when the menstrual cycle is irregular. Specific investigation such as serial ultrasonography may be needed to ascertain the gestational age.

Contraception

Sometimes pregnancy may occur even when oral contraceptive are being used. There may be pregnancy even with an IUCD *in situ*. In the former case duration of pregnancy is difficult to ascertain and with IUCD there might be first trimester abortion.

Past Medical History

Medical disorders such as diabetes mellitus, cardiac problems, hypertension, renal disease, collagen disease and epilepsy may have some deleterious effect on pregnancy.

Gynecological Condition

Conditions such as uterine fibroid, ovarian tumor and genital prolapse are listed as high risk factor. Uterine fibromyoma may lead to abortion in early and mid-pregnancy and premature delivery later on. In early weeks the myoma may undergo red degeneration and presents as acute abdomen. A myoma in lower uterine segment or in cervix can lead to obstructed labor. Postpartum hemorrage is common owing to poor contractility of myometrium.

An ovarian tumor may undergo torsion necessitating emergency ovariotomy. Obstructed labor may result from a tumor impacted at the pouch of Douglus. A prolapsed cervix during pregnancy is engorged and edematous, and is a source of infection leading to abortion. In labor such a cervix refuses to dilate. Recurrent abortion is common with congenital abnormalities of the uterus such as septate uterus, bicornuate uterus, etc. A period of infertility prior to pregnancy is also considered as a risk factor.

Personal history like habit of smoking and consumption of alcohol are likely to cause placental insufficiency. Use of drugs before and after conception in question should be noted.

Family history of multiple pregnancy, fetal abnormality, besides the medical disorders are important risk factor.

Past Obstetric History

Past history of spontaneous abortion and medical termination of pregnancy need special attention. In recurrent abortion whether cervical encirclage was needed or not should be mentioned. The exact duration of pregnancy at which abortions took place should be asked. Development of hypertension with or without proteinuria and the time of onset should be noted.

Duration of gestation at which delivered: Preterm delivery may be repeated. Similarly with history of previous post-dated pregnancy the present pregnancy also may continue beyond term.

Mode of Delivery

Patient with previous caesarean section may require repeat caesarean section. Postpartum hemorrhage and manual removal of placenta are third stage complications which may recur in subsequent deliveries. History of previous still birth, neonatal death, premature delivery and intrauterine growth restriction are other high risk factors. Another important risk factor is Rhesus incompatibility.

❐ PHYSICAL EXAMINATION

On physical examination some risk factors can be identified from the following points:

Height and Weight

A short woman is likely to have a smaller pelvis. Dwarf woman usually have abnormal pelvic configuration. A woman of less than average weight may have lighter babies.

Anemia

Anemia is common in our country. In anemia maternal mortality is very high. Patient may develop right-sided heart failure, intercurrent infection, intrauterine growth restriction due to placental insufficiency and even intrauterine fetal death.

Hypertension

When the diastolic blood pressure is more than 90 mm of Hg hypertension is diagnosed. In a case of essential hypertension pre-eclampsia may superimpose in later weeks of pregnancy. Cardiac problems are usually aggravated in these cases. Hypertension is an important cause of placental insufficiency and hence intrauterine growth restriction, intrauterine fetal death and accidental hemorrhage are common.

Size of the Uterus

Size of the uterus may be smaller or bigger than the period of amenorrhea. Usual causes of smaller size are wrong date, intrauterine growth restriction of fetus, oligohydramnios, intrauterine fetal death, etc. Uterus is bigger in size in multiple pregnancy, polyhydramnios, pregnancy complicated with uterine fibromyoma or ovarian tumor and wrong date.

It seems that the list of the risk factors in pregnancy is a long one. A pregnant woman with any risk factor needs regular check-up and consultation with expert obstetrician is warranted. She should be advised confinement in a big hospital well-equipped with maternity and pediatric departments.

chapter 20

Examination of Lump Abdomen

With a lump in abdomen patient's usual complaint is swelling. Swelling may be associated with pain and other gynecological complaints such as menorrhagia or irregular vaginal bleeding. Pain may accompany an inflammatory swelling as in acute tubo-ovarian mass or in chocolate cyst of ovary or in malignant ovarian tumor. Benign neaoplastic tumors are usually painless. A benign ovarian cyst when undergoes torsion is painful. Menorrhagia is common with uterine fibromyoma and when the surface of a submucous myoma is ulcerated or infected there may be irregular vaginal bleeding with heavy bleeding in between.

Patient should be asked when she first felt the swelling. In case of a painless swelling the patient may not be aware of it. It may be a slow growing tumor and usually remains unnoticed. A painful tumor is noticed early and the patient is aware of its rate of growth. A fast growing painful tumor is likely to be malignant.

Before examination the patient is asked to evacuate her bladder. Lying flat on her back on the examination table abdomen is exposed from xiphisternum to pubic region. Legs should be slightly flexed. Location of the lump is noticed in relation to the four quadrant of the abdomen. A lump of pelvic origin is usually restricted to the infraumbilical region. Lump in the midline is likely to be of

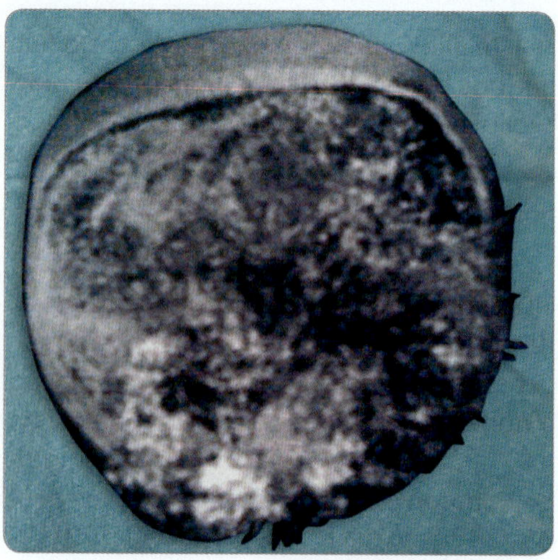

Fig. 1: Dermoid cyst of ovary with hair

uterine origin and lump arising from ovaries and fallopian tubes are restricted to one side. Tubo-ovarian mass or chocolate cysts are present on lateral aspect of the uterus. A benign ovarian cyst, which is mobile, tends to occupy a midline position. Size of the lump may vary greatly. Sometimes an ovarian cyst may attain enormous size and fill up the whole of the abdomen. Shape of the lump is difficult to ascertain abdominally. Surface of the lump can be determined. An ovarian cyst is usually spherical while an uterine lump due to fibromyoma may be regular or irregular in feeling. Bilateral malignant ovarian tumor is irregular in outline. Painful lumps are tender on palpation. Malignant ovarian tumor, chocolate cyst of ovary, tubo-ovarian mass are tender. Similarly twisted ovarian cyst is also tender. Uterine fibromyoma is mobile from side to side, benign ovarian cyst is freely mobile in all directions, but tubo-ovarian mass, chocolate cyst of ovary and malignant ovarian tumor are not mobile. In case of pregnancy of mid-trimester Braxton-Hicks contraction is felt on palpation and fetal parts are palpable. To complete palpation of the abdomen, liver and spleen should be palpated and noted if enlargement is found.

Free peritoneal fluid is present in advanced malignancy. Shifting dullness is useful to exclude fluid collection in the gutters. Whereas fluid thrill is present when peritoneal cavity is mostly filled with ascitic fluid. Sometimes with huge ovarian cyst it may be difficult to differentiate between ovarian cyst and ascites. In ascites there is tympanatic sound on percussion in the midline as the bowel floats in the fluid, whereas in ovarian cyst it is dull on percussion in the midline. In that case tympanatic sound is elicited in the flanks. Sometimes tympanatic sound is present over a lump if bowel is adherent to it as in malignant ovarian tumor or in a lump of tubercular origin.

On auscultation fetal heart sound is heard she is pregnant and duration of pregnancy is 24 weeks or more and uterine soufflé may be present in large uterine fibromyoma also. Bowel sounds may be ausculted over the lump if bowels are adherent to it.

In case of severe pelvic infection following septic abortion or puerperal infection lumps may be felt along the lateral pelvic wall. Swelling may be unilateral or bilateral and it is usually retroperitoneal in origin. These inflammatory lumps are tender and usually associated with rise of temperature and tachycardia. Patient is with toxic look and of ill health. It may suppurate and form a discharging sinus.

Pelvic lump of less than 12 weeks of pregnancy size is not palpable per abdomen. These can be revealed by bimanual examination. Some pelvic lump may extend downwards and fill the pouch of Douglas. Then the lump is felt behind the examining fingers in vagina. Attempt should be made to find out whether it is cystic or solid. Sometimes ovarian cyst may be impacted in the cul-de-sac or a posterior cervical fibromyoma may extend downwards in similar manner.

In any case of pelvic lump rectal examination should be performed. Rectal examination reveals relation of the rectum with the lump. In case of a lump arising from the sacrum examining finger will be anterior to the lump. That lump is usually hard, arising from pelvic bone. Condition of the rectal mucosa should be examined whether it is freely mobile or not. Presence of nodule in pouch of Douglas can be easily felt by rectal examination. Presence of nodule in the pouch of Douglas in case of ovarian tumor indicates secondary metastasis.

❐ INVESTIGATION

In routine blood examination leukocytosis, high erythrocytic sedimentation rate (ESR) indicates presence of infective lump. In malignant tumor also ESR is high.

Among special investigations ultrasonography is helpful to determine the origin of the lump, its size and extent, whether the lump is solid, cystic or variegated in appearance. More sophisticated devices such as CT scan and MRI can determine more details of the lump. These are specially helpful in cases of malignant tumor.

Cytological study of ascitic fluid for malignant cells should be carried out in suspected cases of malignancy.

Vulval Swelling

Vulval swelling may be traumatic, inflammatory or neoplastic. Traumatic swelling is usually following a fall resulting in hematoma formation. In young girl it may be due to sexual abuse also. A hematoma is painful, may be at any place and of any size. Sometimes a hematoma may extend upwards.

On examination of the patient general conditions such as pulse, blood pressure and degree of pallor should be noted. On local examination site, size and extent of the hematoma should be ascertained. To determine upward

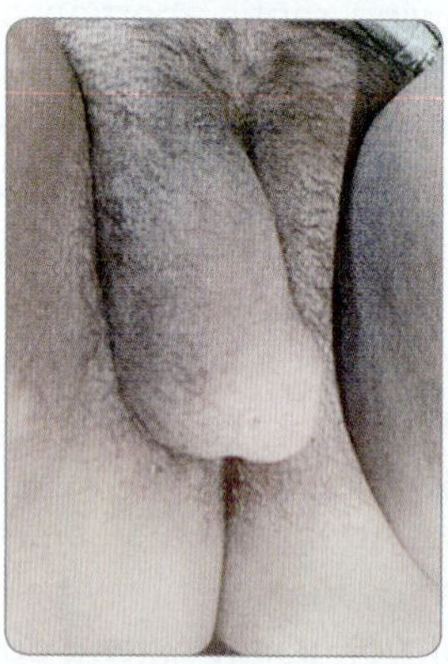

Fig. 2: Lipoma of right labia majora

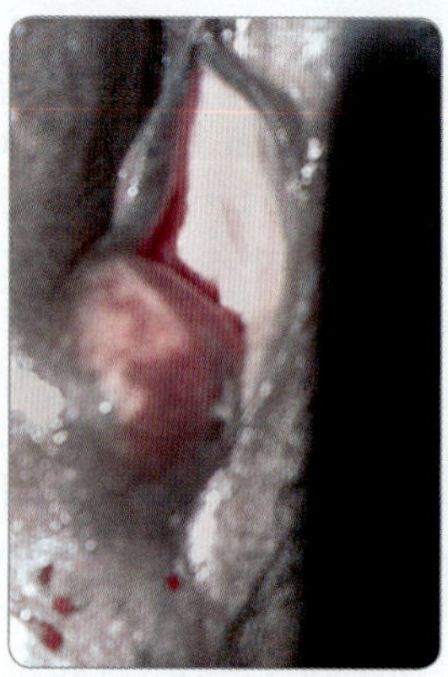

Fig. 3: Bartholin cyst

extension vaginal examination is needed. Swelling of the vaginal wall and its extension upwards determine the extent of the hematoma. Examination under anesthesia particularly in young and nulliparous women is helpful to determine the upward extension.

Acute infection of the Bartholin gland and Bartholin abscess result in painful enlargement in the posterior part of labia. The gland is inflamed with accumulation of exudate inside. The opening of the duct may be blocked. Accumulated exudate suppurate and form abscess. It may burst at any point and pus comes out. Besides Bartholin cyst there may be other inclusion cyst in the anterior aspect of labia. These cysts when inflamed become painful and tender.

Lipoma of vulva is soft, painless swelling of any size. It may even be pedunculated. Other swellings seen in vulva are condyloma acuminata, condyloma lata, granuloma and carcinoma.

Malignant disease of vulva is mostly a disease of elderly age group. Usual presenting symptoms are swelling, ulceration and pruritus. Depending upon the site of involvement patient complains of difficulty in urination. Occasionally there may be bleeding from the lesion. The commonest site is labia majora but in labia minora, clitoris and perineum also the lesion may originate.

❐ DIFFERENTIAL DIAGNOSIS

Full Bladder

It is customary to empty the urinary bladder before gynecological examination. But with chronic retention of urine the bladder may remain full.

- It is a midline suprapubic swelling
- Margins are well defined
- Cystic on palpation and feel the urge to micturate on pressure
- Disappear after catheterization.

Pregnancy

- Period of amenorrhea
- Midline swelling soft in consistency
- Fetal parts may be palpable
- Braxton-Hicks contraction presents
- External ballotment elicited
- On vaginal examination
  - Internal ballotment present
  - Cervix soft
- Ultrasonography – confirms pregnancy.

Ovarian Tumor

- Menstrual history is normal

- May be cystic, solid or of variegated feeling
- Margins are well defined, benign tumors are freely mobile
- Vaginal examination:
  - Uterus felt separately from the tumor
- Ultrasonography confirms diagnosis.

Uterine Fibromyoma

- Menorrhagia or irregular bleeding
- Swelling is firm
- Surface smooth or irregular
- Mobile from side to side
- Vaginal examination
  - Uterine swelling
  - Cervix firm in consistency
  - Cervix moves with movement of the tumor
- Ultrasonography confirms diagnosis.

Adenomyosis

- Menorrhagia with severe dysmenorrhea
- Suprapubic lump
- Regular with smooth surface
- Firm
- On vaginal examination
  - Uterine swelling
  - Cervix firm
  - May be associated with pelvic endometriosis
- Ultrasonography confirms diagnosis.

Tubo-ovarian Mass

- History of pain abdomen
- Recent history of delivery, abortion or medical termination of pregnancy
- Menorrhagia or irregular bleeding with dysmenorrhea of congestive type
- Occasional fever with pain
- Cystic swelling
- Not mobile, tender
- Abnormal vaginal discharge.

On Vaginal Examination

- Uterus may be felt separately or,
- May be attached to the uterus
- Tender fornices
- Cystic, non-mobile lump, tender.

Ultrasonography

- May reveal complex cystic lump.

Endometriosis

- Dysmenorrhea
- Menorrhagia, epimenorrhagia
- Infertility
- Pelvic pain
- Dyspareunia
- Lower abdominal pain
- Pain during defecation.

Vaginal Examination

- Pelvic tenderness
- Nodules in pouch of Douglas
- Uterus fixed
- Bilateral cystic lump.

Ultrasonography

- USG is helpful in diagnosis
- Laparoscopy can confirm the diagnosis.

chapter

21 Menstrual Abnormality

Menstrual abnormality is another common presenting symptom in gynecology. The following points are of importance to note:

Age

Correct age of the patient should be noted. Different abnormalities are common in different age group.

Pattern of Abnormality

The first thing to note is whether the menstrual cycle is short, normal or delayed. The exact interval of the cycle should be enquired. Flow may be scanty or heavy. Normally menstrual blood is liquid. Passage of clot indicates heavy bleeding. There may be prolonged period with scanty or heavy bleeding.

Duration of Abnormality

For how long she is having abnormality. Enquiry should be made whether the abnormality started abruptly or gradually over a period of few months. History of previous menstruation prior to the present abnormality should be asked. Association of pain or other symptom should be enquired.

Menstrual abnormalities are only symptoms of some underlying disease processes. Every attempt should be made to discover the disease for proper diagnosis and subsequent management. The common abnormalities are:

Menorrhagia

Menorrhagia means excessive bleeding during menstruation, the cycle remaining normal. Excessive bleeding may be in amount or duration of bleeding or both.

Menorrhagia may be due to several organic diseases. Sometimes there may be excessive bleeding without any demonstrable organic or hematological condition. This type of bleeding is known as functional uterine bleeding or dysfunctional uterine bleeding. Menorrhagia in young girls is usually of this type, known as puberty menorrhagia. Dysfunctional uterine bleeding may be preceded by a short period of amenorrhea and the cycle is anovulatory. There may be heavy bleeding of short duration or bleeding may be heavy or moderate in amount and prolonged. The later is due to irregular shedding, or may be due to persistence of the corpus luteum function preventing complete disintegration of endometrium during menstruation.

Other common causes of menorrhagia are uterine fibromyoma, adenomyosis, endometriosis, endometrial carcinoma, cervical erosion, etc. Some pathological conditions of pelvis also cause menorrhagia. Pelvic inflammatory disease, tubo-ovarian mass, hydrosalpinx, pelvic abscess, pelvic tuberculosis are the conditions which increase pelvic vascularity and lead to menorrhagia. Endocrine disorders such as early cases of thyrotoxicosis, hypothyroidism and acromegaly in its early stage causes menorrhagia. Blood disorders such as thrombocytopenic purpura, hemoglobin E disease may cause increase blood loss during menstruation.

Some medical conditions cause heavy bleeding during the period. These include cardiac failure, chronic nephritis, pulmonary tuberculosis, etc.

Psychosomatic disturbance may lead to menorrhagia, though temporarily.

Polymenorrhea or Epimenorrhea

In polymenorrhea the cycle is altered but maintains a regularity. The menstrual cycle may be of 15–21 days. The short cycle may be associated with a heavy bleeding phase. If the bleeding is both frequent and heavy it is called epimenorrhagia. It may occur at any age. It may be constitutional from onset of menstruation. Commonly seen following abortion or delivery.

Metrorrhagia

This is inter-menstrual irregular bleeding, may be associated with normal menstrual cycle and normal amount of bleeding. There is usually local cause of the irregular bleeding. Bleeding may be due to ulceration of vagina and cervix, cervical carcinoma, carcinoma endometrium, carcinoma vagina, ulcerated submucus fibromyoma of uterus, cervical mucus polyp or fibromyomatous polyp. Bleeding at the time of ovulation, i.e. at the middle of the cycle is not uncommon. It may occur every month and lasts for few hours. Again there may be premenstrual spotting for few days before onset of bleeding phase.

Menometrorrhagia

In this condition there is heavy bleeding which is irregular. Bleeding may be prolonged too.

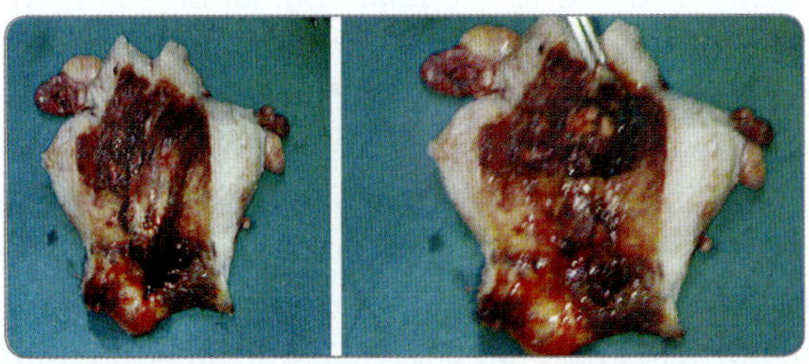

Fig. 1: Cut-section of uterus showing trophoblastic tumor (benign) with polyp formation (left); same specimen showing the lesion involving the cervix (right)

Oligomenorrhea

Oligomenorrhea means infrequent period, the cycle being of more than 35 days. Oligomenorrhea is usually associated with reduced or scanty blood loss.

❐ EXAMINATION OF THE PATIENT

In a women with abnormal menstruation thorough physical examination including complete gynecological examination is carried out.

In general examination presence of anemia and jaundice should be noted. Systemic and gynecological examinations are performed to rule out presence of any organic condition causing the bleeding. In dysfunctional uterine bleeding no organic cause of bleeding can be demonstrated. Palpation of abdomen may reveal tenderness over lower abdomen indicating presence of pelvic inflammation. Tenderness over right iliac fossa may be due to chronic appendicitis. To exclude this condition opinion of a general surgeon may be required. A lump in the suprapubic region may be due to uterine fibromyoma. In that case the lump is in midline, firm and it is usually mobile. It may be regular or irregular in outline and when associated with endometriosis mobility is restricted and bilateral tenderness can be elicited.

Vagina and cervix should be inspected for any ulcerative lesion over it. Ulceration may be a malignant lesion. Cervicitis and erosion of cervix are common conditions. In acute cervicitis the cervix is edematous enlarged and tender. It is an extension of endocervicitis. The cervix is velvety in appearance, red in color owing to increased vascularity, usually covered with mucus discharge. There may be mucus cyst known as nabothian cyst. Erosion is another condition which is usually a consequence of chronic cervicitis. Erosion of cervix is characterized by red granular surface with well-defined margins. Erosion may be simple flat erosion or papillary erosion. Sometimes the ulcer may be tuberculous or even malignant. In suspected cases smear should be taken for culture and sensitivity and for Pap staining.

In bimanual examination the first thing to do is to determine the size of the uterus. Uterus may be enlarged due to pregnancy-related condition such as incomplete abortion, missed abortion or retained product conception. All these conditions give rise to irregular vaginal bleeding which may often be heavy. Uterine fibromyoma and adenomyosis is difficult to distinguish by bimanual examination. But with multiple fibromyoma the uterus is enlarged and of irregular shape. In choriocarcinoma uterus is enlarged and is usually soft in texture. Next the adnexae are palpated. Adnexae are tender in pelvic inflammatory disease. A lump lateral or posterolateral to the uterus may be from chronic infection forming a tubo-ovarian mass. Chocolate cyst of ovaries is another condition where cystic lump is felt, tender and not mobile. Sometimes chronic ectopic pregnancy may form a lump there. This is also tender with restricted mobility. Ovarian cysts are usually not tender but mobile. A definite gap in felt between the uterus and the cyst. A malignant tumor of the ovary is usually fixed and tender.

❐ INVESTIGATIONS

As a first step in evaluation of a woman with abnormal vaginal bleeding routine blood test is done. This includes estimation of hemoglobin concentration, total RBC count, total WBC count and differential leukocytic count. These findings indicate degree of anaemia and presence of infection in pelvis or any where in the body. To exclude bleeding diathesis platelet count, bleeding time, coagulation time should be estimated. Sometimes complete coagulation profile may be needed. In some cases hematological consultation is required. Thyroid profile should be carried out particularly in goitre endemic area to diagnose hyper or hypothyroidism. Random blood sugar estimation gives an idea of the glycemic status of the woman. If random blood sugar is high fasting and postprandial blood sugar should be done to exclude diabetes mellitus. Two-hour oral glucose tolerance test (OGTT) with 75 g of glucose is a sensitive test to confirm glycemic status of the patient.

To exclude pregnancy complication urine examination for β-human chorionic gonadotropin (β-hCG) is helpful and in suspected cases of chorionepithelioma serum β-hCG level should be estimated for confirmation.

Pelvic ultrasonography plays an important role for evaluation of enlarged uterus and pelvic lump. Transvaginal ultrasonography is more informative for evaluation of pelvic pathology, than transabdominal route. In enlarged uterus ultrasonography can detect whether there is retained product of conception, fibromyoma or adenomyosis. Evaluation of endometrial thickness owing to endometrial hyperplasia or presence of endometrial polyp can be determined with accuracy. Computed tomography (CT) or magnetic resonance imaging (MRI) is rarely needed. These are helpful in suspected cases of pelvic malignancy.

Dilatation and curettage (D and C) is a diagnostic procedure. It is an operative procedure and is performed in operation theatre under general anesthesia. Alternatlvely endometrial biopsy or endometrial sampling is an office procedure. One of these procedures is essential to evaluate a woman with abnormal bleeding who are at greater risk of developing endometrial hyperplasia, endometrial polyp or endometrial carcinoma. In D and C the cervix of the uterus is dilated with cervical dilators and endometrium is curetted out with the help of endometrial curette or uterine curette of appropriate size. While in endometrial sampling cervical dilatation is not necessary. Different varities of fine endometrial biopsy curette are available for this purpose. With the help of such a curette few strips of endometrium can be taken out and sent for histopathological examination. To be more precise in selecting the area for biopsy hysteroscopy assisted curettage is more valuable and is a preferred technique nowadays.

Amenorrhea

Amenorrhea means absence of menstruation. A girl gets her first menstruation, menarche by 10–16 years of age. In India the mean age is estimated to be 13.5 years. Different factors such as genetic, environment, social class and nutrition contribute to the age of menarche. Nutrition is an important factor to consider. Obese girls are said to have menarche earlier than thin girls.

Amenorrhea may be due to some physiological conditions such as pregnancy, before puberty, during lactation and after menopause. Amenorrhea is of two types—primary amenorrhea and secondary amenorrhea.

Primary amenorrhea is defined as non-attainment of menarche by 16 years of age or who at any age has never gets menstruations. Secondary amenorrhea refers to cessation of menstruation in a girl/woman who had normal menstruation previously.

Causes of Amenorrhea

In prepubertal stage and after menopause absence of menstruation is the rule. Age of menarche varies and sometimes it may be delayed. If menarche is not attained even by 18 years of age the girl should be examined and cause is to be ascertained for proper treatment. A woman in reproductive age group, having amenorrhea one should suspect pregnancy, unless proved otherwise. In early weeks of pregnancy examination of urine for β-hCG is confirmatory. Period of amenorrhea during breastfeeding varies. During lactation ovulation is suppressed by increased blood level of prolactin, secreted by anterior pituitary. Although the usual period of lactational amenorrhea is about 6 months, patient may have resumption of menstruation even after 6 weeks of delivery.

A woman usually attains her menopause by the age of 45–50 years, but it may occur early also. Menopause is the final cessation of menstruation. It is due to loss of ovarian function.

Pathological Causes of Primary Amenorrhea

Congenital–Certain congenital abnormalities cause amenorrhea as:

Cryptomenorrhea or concealed menstruation: This condition results from retention of menstrual blood. It is commonly due to non-canalization of the lower end of the genital tract or imperforated hymen. This is actually not a case of primary amenorrhea. This condition is characterized by cyclical pain coinciding with each menstruation.

In some girls the uterus may be congenitally absent or hypoplastic. In extreme cases uterus may be represented by a fibromuscular nodule only. Vagina may be normal or non-canalized. Ovarian functions are usually normal and secondary sexual characters are normal.

Gonadal dysgenesis is due to chromosomal abnormality. There is primary ovarian aplasia with streak ovaries. In such cases primary amenorrhea is associated with poorly-developed secondary sex characters. Turner's syndrome is of this variety. Other congenital defects are hermophroditism, hypogonadism, pituitary dwarfism, etc. Systemic diseases such as pelvic tuberculosis or pulmonary tuberculosis in infancy or early childhood may cause primary amenorrhea.

Secondary Amenorrhea

Secondary amenorrhea also may be due to obstruction in the lower genital tract, developed secondarily due to fibrosis. Cervical stenosis may result from fibrosis following extensive cautory or following amputation of cervix. Similarly

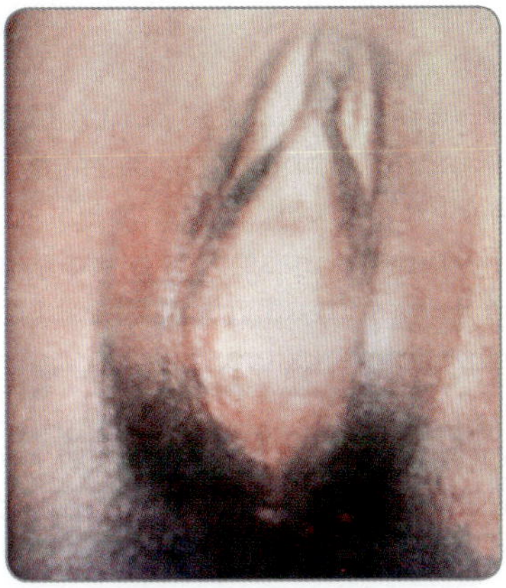

Fig. 2: Cryptomenorrhea with bulging hymen

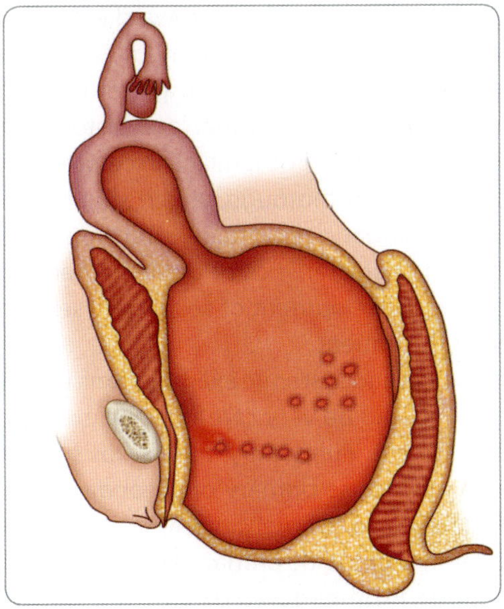

Fig. 3: Cryptomenorrhea, menstrual blood collected in vagina

endometrium may be destroyed following repeated curettage and endometrial tuberculosis. Asherman's syndrome develops intrauterine adhesion or synechie which may obliterate the uterine cavity resulting in amenorrhea. Synechie develops secondary to postpartum or postabortal curettage, manual removal of placenta, etc. Other conditions such as hysterectomy, radiation, severe postpartum or postabortal infection also result in amenorrhea.

Some endocrine disorders such as polycystic ovarian syndrome, Chusing's syndrome, thyroid disorders, hyperprolactinemia also lead to secondary amenorrhea.

Examination of a Case of Amenorrhea

A thorough, systematic examination of the whole body is needed in the initial evaluation of the patient.

Height of the patient should be taken in centimeter and noted in the case note. Dwarfism is an important finding in certain condition like pituitary dwarfism. Weight is taken in kilogram and correlated with height according to the height-weight chart. Body mass index (BMI), an important parameter of nutritional status is calculated by dividing weight in kilogram by height in metersquare, and it is expressed in kilogram per square meter. Normal BMI is around 22.

Hair distribution is another feature to note carefully. One should know the normal hair distribution pattern in female. Abnormal distribution like hair on face, in upper lip, low temporal hair line, hair in chest and around the areola are abnormal. Similarly body hairs also may be coarse, dark black and excessive. Peculiar pattern of hair at the upper margin of mons veneris is important to note. In female pattern there is usually no upward extension whereas in male pattern upward extension in the midline may be there. In case of abnormal hair growth enquiry should be made about pattern of hair growth in other female members of the family like mother and sisters. Because the type of hair growth may be constitutional or familial. Excessive hair growth indicates high androgenic activity. Then thorough search should be made to evaluate the development of secondary sex organs. Development of breast, vulva, vagina, appearance and characteristics of pubic hair and axillary hair should be examined and noted. Development of secondary sex characters should be co-related with age of the patient.

Next is general physical and systemic examinations which should be carried out methodically. One should be very careful while examining the respiratory system and nervous system. Pulmonary tuberculosis is still not uncommon in our country which may cause primary or secondary amenorrhea. Similarly intracranial disorders may lead to amenorrhea.

Pelvic examination in a girl with primary amenorrhea is better performed under general anesthesia. An imperforated hymen leading to cryptomenorrhea is diagnosed by the presence of bulging membrance at the introitus.

Many a times it may not be possible to do vaginal examination due to narrow introitus. In that case per rectum examination is performed. Index finger of the well-lubricated gloved hand is introduced gently inside vagina or rectum, as the case may be and attempt is made to palpate the uterus, while gently pressing the suprapubic region with the other hand. If the uterus is absent it is usually replaced by a fibrotic nodule in the midline. Then the adnaxa are palpated to exclude any cystic or solid mass there, which may be due to ovarian tumor.

In case of lower vaginal atresia an elongated cystic swelling is felt anterior to the finger in rectum. This is hematocolpos resulting from collection of blood from the menstruating uterus. Very rarely uterus may also be enlarged-hematometra, with or without bilateral cystic swelling in pelvis representing hematosalpinx.

❐ INVESTIGATION

Complete blood examination to detect hemoglobin concentration, total RBC count, WBC count, differential leukocytic count is done as routine.

In some cases physical examination may not be sufficient to diagnose Miillerian abnormalities. In these cases pelvic ultrasonography or magnetic resonance imaging (MRI) is helpful. Miillerian abnormality is usually associated with abnormalities of urinary system. An intravenous pyelography should be done in these cases. Karyotyping or chromosomal analysis is needed to confirm if any chromosomal abnormality is suspected.

With normal physical findings if diagnosis is difficult hormone assay is advisable. Hormones, particularly follicle stimulating hormone (FSH), luteinizing hormone (LH), thyroid hormone, ovarian steroids and adrenal cortical hormone assay is done when necessary.

More invasive modern techniques such as laparoscopy and hysteroscopy are helpful for diagnosis of uterine and/or ovarian abnormalities.

chapter

22 Menopausal Problems

Menopause is permanent cessation of menstruation following loss of ovarian function. Surgical menopause follows bilateral oophorectomy with or without removal of uterus.

Perimenopause is a period immediately prior to menopause and at least 12 months after menopause. Post-menopause begins after a period of 12 months of cessation of menstruation.

Menopause is a period of transition from reproductive to non-reproductive period. Menopause occurs at around 50 years of age. This age is thought to be influenced by genetics. It has no relation with social or nutritional status of the woman. Along with this transition effect of ageing influences the physical, psychological and sexual activity of women. For many individual effects of ageing itself is depressing, though most of them accept it as a change of life. Menopausal transition begins gradually from about mid-forties. Following cessation of ovarian function secretion of ovarian steroid, estrogen becomes negligible and that of progesterone also. As a result level of follicle stimulating hormone (FSH) and lutenizing hormone (LH) remain high in circulation. High level of gonadotropins is thought to be the cause of vasomotor symptoms of menopause.

With increasing longevity of man as a whole women population in the postmenopausal period is also increasing. Here lies the importance of study of menpause, menopausal problems faced by the woman and their effective management.

❒ SYMPTOMS

Amenorrhea is the first symptom which may be preceded by prolonged menstrual cycle with normal or heavy flow. It is not normal to have heavy or irregular bleeding. Menstrual abnormality during this period should be evaluated to determine any associated pathological condition. Some women come with history of amenorrhea with a fear of being pregnant and others want to know if there is any pathology to explain amenorrhea.

Hot flush: It is a disturbing symptom of perimenopausal and menopausal period. There is flushing which is transient and recurrent. Along with flushing there may be sensation of heat over the whole body and particularly over the head, as if hot wind is blowing through the ears, often accompanied by palpitation and followed by sweating. The whole episode may last for 1–2 minutes and may recur several times a day.

Hot flush may be accompanied by feeling of fatigue, irritability, anxiety and mental depression. In mild cases reassurance is sufficient but in severe cases hormone replacement therapy results in resolution of these symptoms in most women.

Vaginal symptoms include dryness, dyspareunia, recurrent vaginal infection and burning urination. Urinary symptoms are dysuria, recurrent urinary tract infection and urge incontenence. Atrophic changes in urethra may lead to urgency and stress incontenence.

Women of perimenopausal period or after menopause may suffer from lack of power of concentration or even there may be loss of memory.

Bone changes during menopause is a concern to the patient and her physician. Osteoporosis is a condition of reduction in the quality of bone. Bones become thin and prone to fracture easily. This is an effect of estrogen deficiency. Hormone replacement therapy may minimize bone loss and prevent osteoporosis. Calcium supplementation is essential. Most of the women are asymptomatic.

On examination, accumulation of fat is noticeable around hip and buttocks. Systematic examination of breast should be carried out. On pelvic examination signs depend upon period of menopause. Changes of genital organs are progressive and hence depend on how long she is having amenorrhea. In case the period of amenorrhea is of short duration findings correspond to the age of the patient which will be different after a prolonged period of amenorrhea. In that case signs of atrophy will be pronounced. Vulva, vagina show signs of progressive atrophy. There is thinning of vaginal mucosa with loss of rugae. Portiovaginalis of cervix is flushed with the vault of vagina. Uterus is felt smaller than normal size.

❐ POSTMENOPAUSAL BLEEDING

Patient may come with history of vaginal bleeding after menopause. Bleeding may be scanty or of moderate amount. There may be only single episode of bleeding or it may be irregular.

The causes among the benign conditions are hormone replacement therapy, atrophic vaginitis, atrophic endometritis, cervical and intrauterine polyp. Among the malignant conditions are carcinoma cervix, carcinoma vagina or carcinoma endometrium.

Hormone replacement therapy may cause regular monthly bleeding but if taken irregularly there may be irregular bleeding. Ovarian malignancy particularly hormone producing ovarian tumors may cause endometrial hyperplasia and irregular vaginal bleeding.

In history taking, care should be taken to elicit history of hormone replacement therapy, if any. How long it is been taken, whether taken regularly or not. After history thorough physical examination is carried out. In abdominal examination attempt should be made to find out any area of tenderness or lump in lower abdomen.

On pelvic examination vulva is inspected for any ulceration. On speculum examination vagina and cervix are inspected. In elderly woman with long standing menopause vagina is usually narrow with thin vaginal mucosa. For speculum examination a small speculum may be needed, and care should be not taken to injure the vaginal wall. In atrophic vaginitis punctate spot will be noticeable over the vaginal mucosa. Cervix may reveal an ulcer or a growth. Pap smear should be taken from the cervix. When there is evident growth or when pap smear report is suspicious cervical biopsy is mandatory. Colposcopy directed biopsy of cervix is more accurate. In any suspicious growth of vulva and vagina biopsy should be taken to exclude malignancy.

In postmenopausal bleeding endometrial sampling or full D and C should be carried out. It is more useful if hysteroscopy aided endometrial sampling is taken. Ultrasonography of lower abdomen and pelvis is helpful in cases of a lump in pelvis.

chapter

23 Excessive Vaginal Discharge

During reproductive period in normal condition normal vaginal discharge keeps the vagina moist. Mucoid discharge from endometrium, cervical glands and fluid exudate from vaginal epithelium, discharge from Bartholin glands, and Skenes tubules constitute the vaginal discharge. It also contains exfoliated vaginal and cervical epithelial cells. Normally the vaginal secretion is acidic. The predominant comensial bacteria in vagina is lactobacillous. Lactogen is deposited in the epithelial cells of vaginal wall. Lactogen is converted to lactic acid, which is responsible for the acidic reaction of vaginal fluid. The pH of normal vagina is lower than 4.5. This acidity prevents bacterial colonization. If due to some reasons like excess of cervical discharge, which is alkaline, diminishes local resistance or presence of foreign body, bacterial growth and hence vaginitis is favored by alteration of vaginal pH. In childhood and long after menopause this protective mechanism is not available in vagina.

White discharge per vagina is a common complaint in gynecological clinic. In majority of cases the cause is local vaginitis or cervicitis. It may be associated with itching vulva, pain and dysuria. Detail history taking and thorough physical examination are sufficient to identify the cause. But sometimes laboratory help may be needed. During history taking the following points should be noted.

Duration of the complaint should be enquired. How long she is having this complaint and whether it is increasing in amount. The amount of discharge can be assumed by the fact, whether she has to use sanitary napkin or not. At the same time enquiry should be made about the timing of discharge in relation to the menstrual cycle. Physiologically vaginal discharge increases post-menstrually and in the mid-cycle period.

In a woman of reproductive age group history of abortion or child birth in recent past should be taken. Association of pain in lower abdomen with discharge is important to note. Pain in lower abdomen indicates chronic pelvic inflammatory disease. Patient may feel pain in vagina and vulva also. Very often discharge is associated with pruritus vulva. Presence of pruritus in vulval region with white discharge point towards monilial or triochomonas infection of lower genital tract.

❒ BACTERIAL VAGINOSIS

Bacterial vaginosis is mainly due to anaerobic bacteria resulting from change of normal bacterial flora of vagina. The discharge is of fishy odor. The discharge thinly coats the vaginal wall. Microscopic examination reveals plenty of pus cells.

Trichomonas Vaginitis

Trichomonas vaginitis is a sexually transmitted disease. Patient complains of vaginal discharge accompanied by itching vagina. The discharge is purulent, profuse and with foul smell. On microscopic examination motile trichomonas vaginalis are in plenty and leukocytes are present.

Monilial Vaginitis

It is a fungal infection caused mostly by candida albicans. Fungal vaginal infection is commonly found during pregnancy and in patients with diabetes mellitus. There is inflammation of vagina associated with extensive pruritus.

On speculum examination vagina is found to be inflammed and smeared with cardy white discharge. There may be sign of scratching over the vulval skin due to intense pruritus. Patient may also complain of burning or soreness or even pain in vulva and vagina, particularly after urination. Gram stain of the discharge reveals budding spore or mycelia of fungus.

Other causes of vaginal discharge may be foreign body inside vagina. In young girls broken parts of toy or even small grain may be sufficient to cause chronic vaginal discharge owing to vaginal infection. Benign growth of uterus like submucus fibromyoma, myomatous polyp may cause vaginal discharge. Benign cervical condition such as cervicitis, cervical erosion and mucus polyp also lead to excessive vaginal discharge. Among the malignant conditions carcinoma cervix and vagina are important to remember. Vaginal discharge due to these conditions are having typical odor.

It is clear that excessive vaginal discharge may be due to various conditions. After history taking methodical vaginal examination is necessary for diagnosis of the condition. On speculum examination the nature of discharge, condition of vagina and cervix are observed and noted in the case sheet. In young girl speculum examination may be performed under general anesthesia. The discharge should be examined microscopically.

For microscopic examination of the discharge a small amount of the discharge is suspended in normal saline. A drop from there is placed on a clean glass slide and covered with a cover slide, and examined under microscope. Normal vaginal secretion reveals exfoliated normal vaginal epithelial cells and few leukocytes. Gram stain is helpful to detect mycelia or budding yeasts of fungal infection.

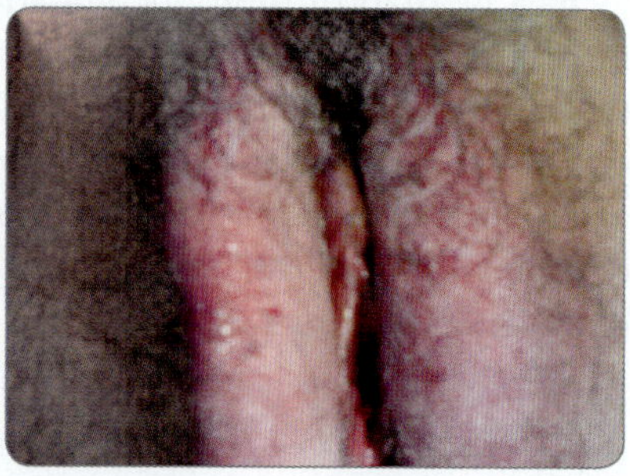

Fig. 1: Acute vulvitis

chapter

24 Infertility

Last few decades have witnessed tremendous improvement in the field of infertility worldwide. It has become a highly sophisticated and specialized discipline within Obstetrics and Gynecology practice. Separate infertility clinic has come-up with facilities for investigation and treatment. Only primary evaluation of the infertile couple will be dealt with here.

Inability to conceive after one year of unprotected coitus is termed as infertility. Two types of infertility are described as – primary infertility in which the woman has not conceived previously and, secondary infertility in which the woman has history of previous pregnancy, which may not end in a live birth. Maximum number of women conceive within 12 months of unprotected coitus. Fertility decreases with age and the decline is more steep after 35 years of age.

❒ HISTORY TAKING

Both the partners should be present during history taking. It is known that in more than 30% of cases male factor is responsible for infertility.

❒ AGE

Age is an important factor in infertile couple. As has been mentioned above fertility in woman declines sharply after 35 years of age, in male this decline is noted after 45 years. Occupation is another factor. So detail occupational history should be taken. Occupational exposure to heat or some chemicals may impair fertility, particularly in male.

Detail history of menstruation is essential. Length of menstrual cycle with its variations should be asked. Irregularity of cycle and period of prolonged amenorrhea, if any, should be noted. Duration of bleeding phase is another factor which needs careful attention from the gynecologist. Women having prolonged bleeding period though may be scanty needs treatment before attempt is made for conception. Menstruation may be associated with pain abdomen. Patient may experience pain before, during or after the bleeding phase. Each one of these has different implication.

In secondary infertility history of previous pregnancy and pregnancy outcome is important to note. Medical termination of pregnancy is very commonly performed to get rid of unwanted pregnancy. Repeated curettage may weaken the endometrium and mild infection during the procedure may lead to tubal block, pelvic adhesion and even uterine synechie, creating problem for future pregnancy. Spontaneous abortion may also have similar effect. In case of delivery of viable fetus duration of pregnancy at the time of delivery, mode of delivery, whether it was live birth or still birth should be enquired. Number pregnancy and pregnancy outcome of each should be noted in the case note chronologically with date and place of delivery. Postpartum or postabortal infection is very common in our country and an important cause of chronic pelvic inflammation and tubal block as a sequel.

Next point to enquire is coital frequency and presence of coital problem. Infrequent coitus particularly non-utilization of the ovulation period is another cause of infertility. Many couple have misconception about the fertile period of the cycle leading to infertility. Regarding coital problem successful penetration and timely ejaculation are to be ensured.

Contraceptives used, its duration, time of stoppage should be enquired. Any problem experienced by the woman is important to note. Pattern of menstruation after stoppage of contraceptives is a useful information.

For the male partner any problem during coitus should be enquired. History of injury in testes, history of surgery particularly hernia repair or operation for hydrocele which may influence spermatogenesis should be noted. Again enquiry should be made of mumps in childhood leading to orchitis. Childhood orchitis destroys the seminiferus tubules and leads to defective spermatogenesis.

Thorough examination of genital organs should be carried out. If any abnormality is detected or suspected help of urologist should be taken for proper evaluation.

The causes of infertility in female are grouped together as:

- Ovulation disorder
- Defect in the fallopian tubes—blockage, peritubal adhesions
- Abnormalities of cervical mucus
- In male abnormalities of semen.

With a view to point out the defect thorough clinical examination is carried out and few laboratory investigations are performed. Physical examination of the patients includes general examination and thorough pelvic examination. In general examination, height and weight are taken, body mass index (BMI) is calculated and noted. Special attention is needed to find out features of thyroid gland dysfunction. Excessive hair growth and other androgenic features are searched for to exclude polycystic ovarian syndrome. On abdominal examination palpation is carried out systematically to find out presence of tender area anywhere in lower abdomen or presence of lump in the suprapubic region. If detected, examination is carried out to determine the location and nature of the lump.

Pelvic examination is carried out in usual manner to exclude any pelvic pathology. Presence of pathological lesion in pelvis, cervix and vagina calls for further evaluation.

❒ LABORATORY INVESTIGATIONS

Laboratory investigations include routine blood examination, VDRL test and urine analysis. Pelvic ultrasonography is done to determine the anatomical status of the pelvic organs, specially the ovaries. Ultrasonography is specially helpful in evaluation of a case with menstrual abnormalities, particularly delayed cycle and cases with amenorrhea.

Investigations are planned to evaluate different causative factors as:

Ovulatory Factor

Ovulatory disorder is responsible for infertility in about one-third of cases. Regular menstrual cycle is thought to be ovulatory one. Otherwise it may be anovulatory or oligo-ovulatory or infrequent ovulation.

Detection of Ovulation

Basal body temperature: This is the easiest and least expensive method. In this method, the woman takes her temperature every morning and record it on a chart. Temperature should be taken before getting out of bed or before drinking anything. Oral temperature should be taken. It should be started from the first day of menstruation. In ovulatory cycle following ovulation there is secretion of progesterone from the corpus luteum. Progesterone is thermogenic and leads to increase of temperature by 0.5°F over the baseline temperature of the luteal phase. Temperature remains elevated giving a biphasic pattern. Biphasic pattern of temperature is characteristic of ovalutory cycle. But sometimes even after ovulation temperature pattern may remain monophasic, that means there is no elevation of temperature even after ovulation. Usually monophasic pattern of temperature is found in anovulatory cycle.

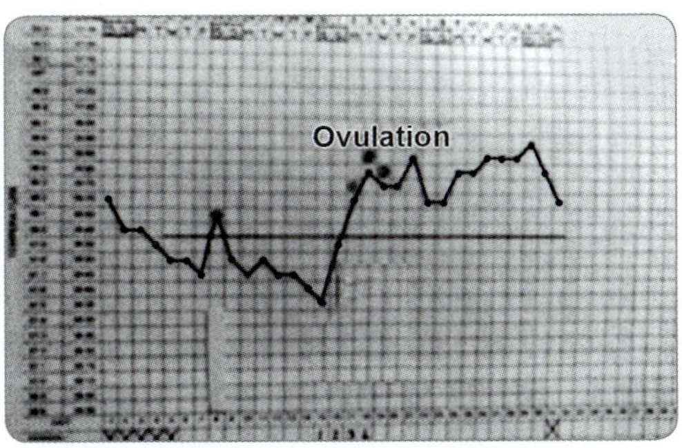

Fig. 1: Basal body temperature chart

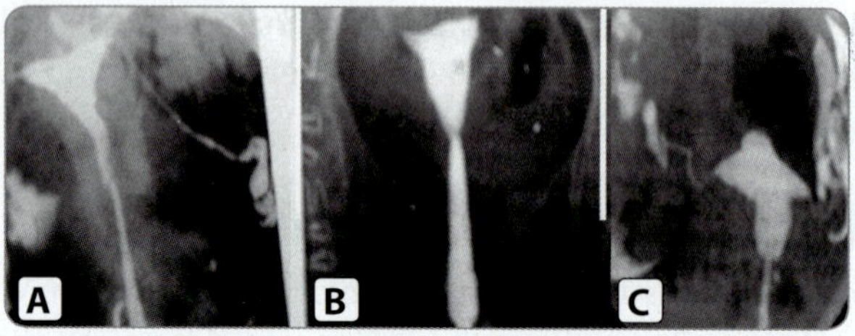

Figs 2A to C: (A) Hysterosalpingography shows bilateral tubal block; (B) Corneal block; (C) Bilateral patent tubes

Midluteal Serum Progesterone: Serum progesterone level of >3 ng/mL on 21st–23rd day of a 28-day cycle confirms ovulation.

Endometrial Biopsy: Evidence of secretory endometrium in endometrial biopsy is confirmatory of ovulation.

Ultrasonography: Serial ultrasonographic study can detect development of dominant follicle and then ovulation. Decrease in follicular size and appearance of fluid in cal-de-sac are taken as evidence of ovulation.

Tubal patency test: Tubal factor is again responsible for about one-third of the cases of female infertility. Tubal block or peritubal adhesions are sequel of pelvic inflammatory disease and endometriosis.

Hysterosalpingography: It is a radiological procedure to detect tubal patency, performed between 7–10 days of menstruation. A water-soluble radio opaque dye is introduced inside the uterus with the help of a canula or a small Foley catheter and radiographs are taken. Usually two radiographs are enough to demonstrate uterine cavity and the tubes. This procedure is contraindicated in presence of vaginitis, cervicitis or pelvic infection and when there is irregular vaginal bleeding.

Laparoscopy: Laparoscopy allows direct visualization of the fallopian tubes, ovaries and pelvic adhesions. Tubal patency may be confirmed by passage of dye like methylene blue through fimbrial opening of the tubes, after the dye is pushed through the cervical canal. This procedure is known as chromopertubation. Another advantage of laparoscope is that adhesions can be removed and in endometriosis appropriate surgery, if needed, can be performed, in the same sitting.

Cervical factor: The quality of cervical mucus and its reaction with sperm is assessed by postcoital test. This test is performed 1 or 2 days before expected date of ovulation (period of high estrogen concentration) and after 2–8 hours of coitus. Cervical mucus is taken out with the help of a long forceps or a tuberculin syringe. Mucus is placed on a clean dry glass slide and covered with a cover slip.

The slide is examined under microscope and number of motile sperm per high power field is counted. Presence of at least five motile sperm per high

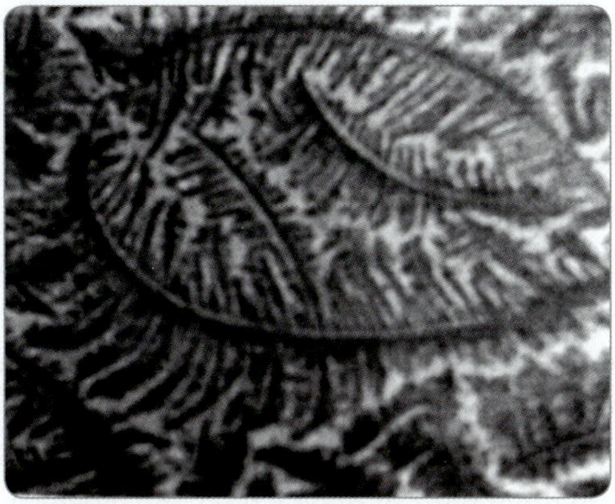

Fig. 3: Fern pattern of cervical mucus

power field is taken as normal. But the utility of PCT as a diagnostic tool in infertility has been questioned by many.

Spinnbarkeit test: This test can be performed to assess the estrogenic effect of cervical mucus. High level of estrogen makes cervical mucus elastic and can be stretched to 8–10 cm when pulled. Mucus is placed on a slide and covered with a cover slide. The cover slide is pulled apart and stretched. After ovulation under the influence is progesterone the cervical mucus become viscous and the thread breaks down.

Fern test: Cervical mucus is dried on a glass slide and examined under microscope. Under microscope characteristic fern pattern is seen. This is due to crystallization of sodium chloride with mucus. Under progesterone effect mucus lacks ferning. Hence absence of ferning indicates ovulation.

Uterine factor: Uterine factors like submucus fibroid and congenital abnormality such as unicornuate uterus, uterine didelphys are associated with infertility. Uterine synechie is another uterine cause of infertility. For diagnosis of these conditions hysterosalpingography is helpful.

❒ SEMEN ANALYSIS

Analysis of husband's semen constitutes measurement of semen volume, assessment of sperm count, sperm motility and morphology of sperm.

Semen analysis should be done after a period of 2–7 days of abstinence. Semen is obtained by masturbation and collected in a wide mouthed dry and clean container. The specimen should reach the laboratory within half-an-hour to one hour of collection. Semen is examined after liquifaction.

Normal semen is gray in color and has opalescent appearance. It has got a peculiar musty odor and viscous in nature. Semen specimen liquefies within 30 minutes of ejaculation.

Volume: Normal volume per ejaculation is about 2–6 mL. Semen is alkaline, the pH ranges from 7.3 to 8.

Sperm count: Sperm count varies widely, even in normal fertile individual. According to WHO, the normal sperm concentration is 20 million/mL or more for spontaneous conception to occur.

Sperm motility: In a normal ejaculation sperm may have 25% rapid progressive motility or 50% rapid and slow progressive motility.

Sperm Morphology: In a normal ejaculate about 30% sperms are of normal morphology with a head, neck, midpiece and tail.

Cellular Elements: Cellular elements present in a normal specimen are sperm precursors, cell from other parts of genital tract and leukocytes.

Oligozoospermia: When sperm count is less than 20 million/mL it is called oligozoospermia. A man should not be considered oligospermic until at least 3 samples are evaluated at an interval of 3 weeks and 3 months.

Azoospermia: It is when the semen sample has no spermatozoa.

Teratozoospermia: It is presence of more than 70% abnormal spermatozoa.

Necrozoospermia: It is when semen sample shows all dead spermatozoa.

them can empty the urinary bladder reposing the cystocele with the help of fingers. Incomplete emptying may lead to accumulation of residual urine, inviting infection. Frequency of micturation results from incomplete emptying and urinary infection. When infection supervene, patients feel pain in lower abdomen and during micturation. Stress urinary incontnence may be present and enquiry should be made of urgency also. Stress incontnence is more common with cystocele or genital prolapse as a whole. Similarly rectocele may lead to incomplete emptying of the rectum which the patient usually complains as constipation.

Vaginal discharge and irregular bleeding result from long standing uterine prolapse and decubitus ulcer. Rarely carcinoma cervix also causes irregular bleeding and discharge from the lesion.

❒ EXAMINATION OF THE PATIENT

Diagnosis of genital prolapse is usually simple. On general examination nothing is specific except that the patients may be anemic or sometimes may be debilitated. On abdominal examination search should be made for any lump and if present needs detail examination.

Physical examination should be performed in dorsal position with the legs flexed. Some gynecologist prefers to perform the examination in Sim's lateral position for ease of doing speculum examination. To begin with vulva, vagina are carefully inspected to identify erosion, ulceration or any other lesions. If such lesions are identified swab should be taken for culture and sensitivity test and biopsy is taken accordingly.

Determination of the extent of prolapse is not difficult in advanced prolapse. In less extent of prolapse it may be difficult to identify its different component particularly on inspection alone. If there is no apparent displacement of uterus the labia are separated to expose the introitus. Patient is asked to strain down or cough forcefully. During straining extent of descent of the pelvic organs are noted and laxity of perineum is also noted. Leakage of urine through the urethral meatus during coughing or straining indicate presence of stress incontinence.

Cystocele can be recognized by a bulging of the anterior vaginal wall and rectocele by a bulging of the posterior vaginal wall. Sim's posterior vaginal speculum is introduced inside vagina. Depressing the speculum posteriorly anterior bulging can be demonstrated well. But visualization of the posterior vaginal wall is difficult with the Sim's speculum. Bulging of the upper part of the posterior vaginal wall represent enterocele. Digital depression of the perineal body while the patient coughs helps to visualize the cystocele and enterocele as well. Bulging of the lower part of the anterior vaginal wall represents urethrocele which usually accompanies cystocele. To detect prolapse of the apex of the vagina after hysterectomy anterior and posterior vaginal walls are retracted and the woman is asked to cough. In presence of prolapse of the apex a protruding mass is observed. Detection of enterocele is not very easy in many cases. To demonstrate enterocele Sim's speculum is withdrawn slowly and the patient is asked to cough. In presence of enterocele the posterior vaginal wall above the speculum will bulge.

Alternatively, rectovaginal examination can be done (Fig. 3). Index finger of the examining hand is kept inside the rectum and the thumb or the middle finger is kept inside the vagina. A rectocele can be differentiated from an enterocele by passing the finger in the rectum into the bulge. In case of rectocele the bulge is at a lower level and limited upwards, whareas in enterocele the bulge is at a higher level and continues upwards. An enterocele is diagnosed on rectovaginal examination by noting the herniated sac. On standing rectovaginal examination a loop of small bowel may be felt between the fingers. Rectovaginal examination is also helpful to detect prolapse of the vault of vagina after hysterectomy.

Descent of the uterus inside vagina can be seen during speculum examination. In advanced degree of prolapse the cervix is seen at or outside the vaginal introitus. There is elongation of the supravaginal portion of the cervix in second degree uterine prolapse. This can be demonstrated by passing an uterine sound. In procedentia whole of the uterus is outside the vaginal introitus. Fingers of the examining hand are placed behind the protruding

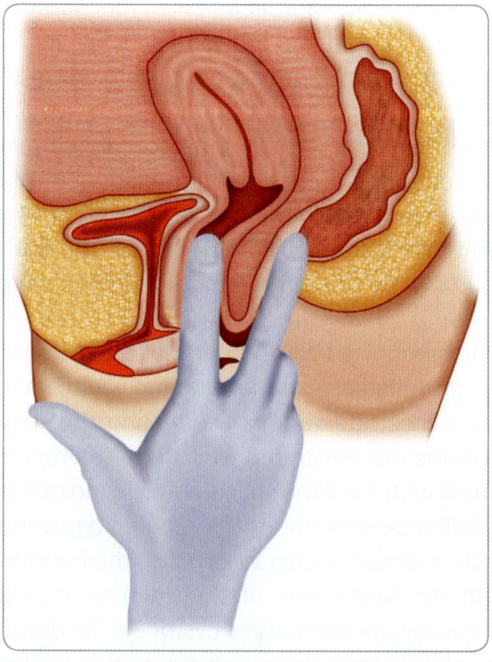

Fig. 3: Rectovaginal examination in enterocele

mass at the level of the introitus and the thumb anteriorly. In procedentia the fundus of the uterus is felt below the grip whereas in second-degree uterine prolapse the uterus is gripped between the fingers. In long-standing prolapse decubitus ulcer may be present over the vaginal wall or the cervix.

At last a careful bimanual vaginal examination is done to exclude presence of any pelvic mass. Careful assessment of the pelvic organ support is made to plan the appropriate operative procedure.

❒ OTHER CONDITIONS WHICH MAY MIMIC GENITAL PROLAPSE

Congenital elongation of cervix, cervical polyp and chronic inversion of uterus.

Congenital Elongation of Cervix

Congenital elongation of the cervix is confined to the vaginal portion of the cervix. The external os may be seen at or outside the introitus. On examination fundus of the uterus is found in its normal position. Vaginal fornices are deep and there is no evidence of cystocele and rectocele.

Rarely inclusion cysts may develop in vagina. Gartner's duct cyst in lower vagina tends to occupy towards the midline in the anterior wall. Anterior and posterior cysts simulate cystocele and rectocele respectively. The cyst can be differentiated from cystocele and rectocele by the findings that there is no vaginal rugae over the tense cyst wall and the cysts are not reducible. Sometimes with fibromyomatous polyp or chronic inversion of uterus patient complains of fullness of vagina and vaginal discomfort. Speculum examination can easily differentiate these from uterine descent.

chapter

26 Fibromyoma of Uterus

Fibromyoma of uterus is the most common benign tumor of female genital tract. Fibromyoma is again known as myoma, fibroid or uterine leomyoma. Most of these remain asymptomatic.

Types

Maximum number of fibromyoma are found in the body of the uterus (corporeal), only few develop in the cervical region. According to position in the uterus fibromyomas are classified into the following types:

Subserous

This type of fibromyoma are found on the outer surface of the uterus. It is again known as subperitoneal. Subserous fibromyoma arises from the outer layers of myometrium. Sometimes it may grow between the layers of broad ligament on the lateral wall of the uterus. Then it is called broad ligament fibromyoma (false or pseudo). True broad ligament fibromyoma arise from the round ligament or from the muscle fibers of blood vessels inside the broad ligament. A subserous fibromyoma may be pedunculated. And may be of very big in size.

Interstitial or Intramural

It grows inside the substance of the myometrium. Intramural variety is the commonest one. When it grows bigger it may become subserus or submucus.

Submucus

This variety of fibromyoma grows beneath the endometrium of the uterus and may project inside the uterine cavity. As a result of the expulsive force of the uterus a submucus tumor may become pedunculated and ultimately polypoidal and remains inside the uterine cavity. In course of time a fibromyomatous polyp may extrude through the cervix. In this process the polyp may lead to chronic inversion of the uterus. Submucous fibromyoma are prone to get ulcerated, infected or sloughed.

Cervical

In cervical region fibromyoma may be single or multiple in number.

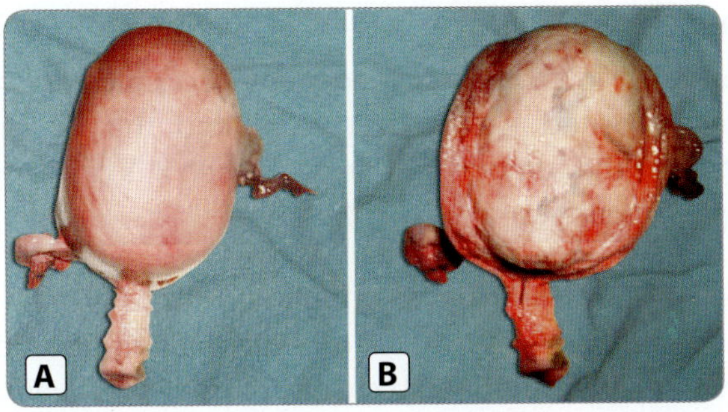

Figs 1A and B: (A) Uniform enlargement of the uterus due to single fibromyoma; (B) The same uterus cut open – big submucus myoma

Cervical fibromyoma may grow in any part of the cervix. It may be supravaginal or in the vaginal portion of the cervix. In vaginal portion it is rare and when grows projects towards the vaginal canal and often become polypoidal.

In supravaginal portion it may be:

Anterior: Cervical fibromyoma growing from the anterior wall pushes the urinary bladder and may cause urinary symptoms.

Posterior: Posterior cervical fibromyoma grows posteriorly and occupies the pouch of Douglas and may grow downwards.

Lateral: Lateral cervical fibromyoma usually grows between the two layers of broad ligaments. These tumors push the ureter laterally.

Central: Central cervical tumor expands the cervix on all sides pushing the body of the uterus upwards.

❐ SECONDARY CHANGES

Different degenerative changes may take place in fibromyoma:

Hyaline Degeneration

This is the most common type of degeneration usually seen in large tumor. Degeneration first starts at the central part which is least vascular. The tumor becomes soft in consistency.

Cystic Degeneration

Following hyaline degeneration there may be liquifaction of the tumor material to from cystic degeneration. The material becomes gelatinous and the tumor looks saggy. This change is common in post-menopausal woman.

Fatty Degeneration

In this type of degeneration fat globules are deposited inside the tumor.

Calcification

Calcification usually follows fatty degeneration. Calcium carbonate and phosphate are deposited within the tumor and the tumor is felt hard. Sometimes whole of the tumor is calcified and then it is called 'womb stone'. It is common in post-menopausal women.

Red Degeneration

Red degeneration usually occurs during pregnancy and puerperium. Partial necrosis occurs inside the tumor with chance of partial recovery. It is known as necrobiosis. On naked eye examination of cut-section shows partly red areas of raw-meat appearance and fishy in odor. Color is due to hemolysis of blood. The cause is thought to be vascular in origin.

Atrophy

Atrophy of the fibromyoma is thought to be due to diminished vascularity.

Necrosis

Necrosis is mostly central. Sometime the whole tumor may be effected.

Infection

Infection is more common in submucus fibromyoma, usually after child birth or abortion. An ulcerated area of a submucus fibromyoma may get infected and slough out.

Vascular Changes

Some vascular changes like dilatation of the vessels or lymphatics may occur.

Malignant Change

Rarely sarcomatous change may occur in a benign fibromyoma.

Changes in the Pelvis Caused by Fibromyoma of Uterus

The changes brought about in the pelvis depend on the number and size of the tumor.

Uterus

A moderate size submucus fibroid causes uniform enlargement of the uterus (Fig. 2). Multiple tumors of different types and sizes make the uterus enlarged and distorted. It may fill the abdomen upto umbilicus or above. Cavity of uterus elongates and gets distorted. Myohyperplasia is almost constant.

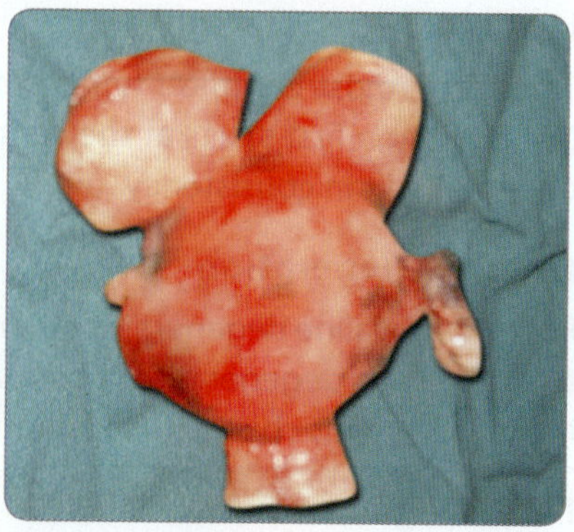

Fig. 2: Multiple fibromyoma of uterus

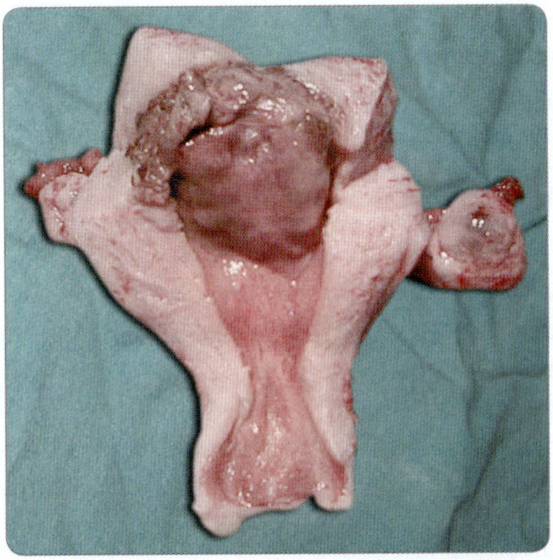

Fig. 3: Degenerated submucus fibromyoma of uterus

Endometrium is usually hyperplastic, but endometrium overlying a submucus fibromyoma is thinned-out and may be ulcerated. Vessels are engorged.

Fallopian Tubes

Fallopian tubes show signs of inflammation. Uterine opening of the tubes may be blocked by a fibromyoma situated at the cornual end of the uterus.

The Ovaries

The ovaries may be enlarged with multiple cysts.

Ureter

Ureter may be displaced by the broad ligament fibromyoma. A pseudo broad ligament fibromyoma may push the ureter laterally, whereas a true broad ligament tumor may push it medially. Pressure effect of a benign tumor is very rare, but sometimes pressure over the ureter may cause hydroureter and even hydronephrosis.

Endometriosis

Endometriosis and/or adenomyosis may be associated with fibromyoma.

Endometrial Carcinoma

Uterine fibromyoma has no definite correlation with endometrial carcinoma.

❒ PRESENTING SYMPTOMS

Majority of women remain asymptomatic. Asymptomatic fibromyoma are incidental findings of ultrasonography of pelvis or laparotomy done for some other indications.

Symptoms depend on the site and size of the tumor. Subserous tumor produces no symptom unless it is large. Intramural and submucus fibromyoma produces more symptoms.
Usual symptoms are:

Menstrual Abnormality

Menorrhagia

Menorrhagia is the most common variety of menstrual irregularity. With passage of time blood loss increases with passage of clot. Causes of menorrhagia are:
- Increased bleeding surface
- Endometrial hyperplasia
- Increased vascularity and pelvic congestion
- Impaired contractility of uterus due to presence of fibromyoma.

Metrorrhagia or Irregular Bleeding

Metrorrhagia is due to ulceration of a submucus or polypoidal fibromyoma, associated carcinoma endometrium also may cause irregular bleeding.

Dysmenorrhea

Congestive dysmenorrhea may be due to associated pelvic congestion. Uterine contractility to extrude a submucus myoma or to expel a myomatus polyp through the cervical canal causes spasmodic dysmenorrhea.

Infertility

Presence of fibromyoma of uterus may cause infertility. Different causes such as impaired sperm transport, defective implantation are attributed for inability to conceive.

Besides infertility presence of fibromyoma during pregnancy may lead to repeated abortion, premature delivery, abnormal presentation, intrauterine growth restriction and increased incidence of postpartum hemorrhage.

Anemia, general debility may be there due to prolonged episode of menorrhagia or irregular vaginal bleeding.

❐ ON EXAMINATION

General Examination

Anemia is usually present.

Abdominal Examination

Small tumor is not palpable per abdomen, only when the size of the uterus is bigger than 12 weeks of pregnancy size it becomes palpable. When palpable the lump is firm in consistency.
- Surface may be smooth or irregular depending on the number of fibromyoma.
- Margins are well-defined can be moved from side to side.

Bimanual Examination

Bimanual examination reveals an enlarged uterus, firm in consistency and with irregular outline. The lump moves with movement of the cervix and the uterus cannot be felt separately. These last two findings confirm that the lump is of uterine origin. Rectal examination confirms the findings of bimanual examination.

Laboratory Investigations

- Complete blood examination to determine the degree of anemia.
- Ultrasonography of pelvis is a useful procedure to confirm the diagnosis of fibromyoma. Vaginal ultrasonography can detect the ovarian pathology, if any, precisely, thereby can differentiate a subserous myoma or a pedunculated subserous myoma from an ovarian tumor.

Magnetic resonance imaging (MRI) is more precise but not always needed for diagnosis of fibromyoma.

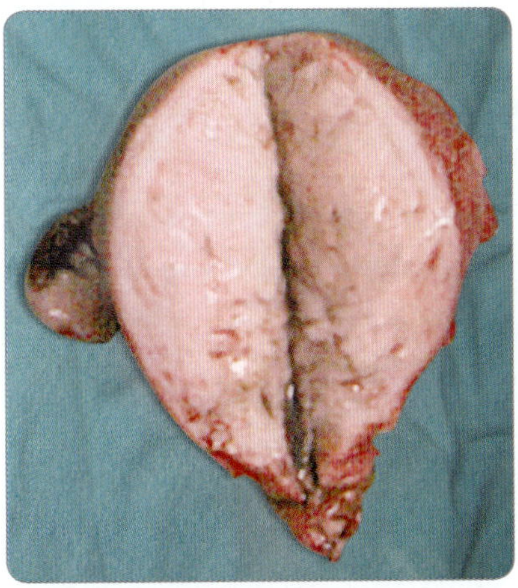

Fig. 4: Adenomyosis of uterus

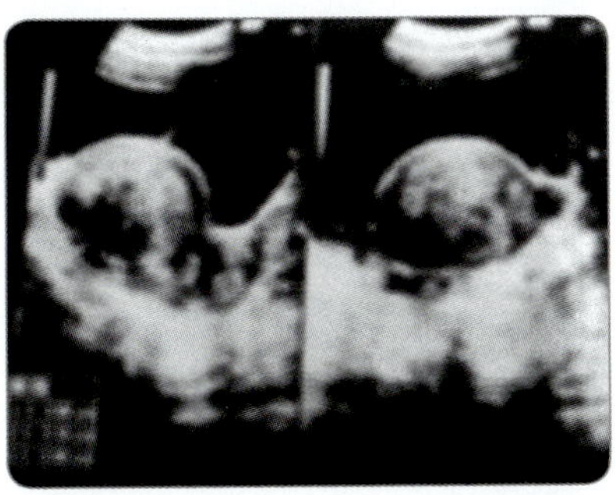

Fig. 5: Ultrasonography showing a fibromyoma

Laparoscopy

Laparoscopy is useful in cases of fibromyoma of uterus associated with infertility or endometriosis. It is also helpful to know the condition of the fallopian tubes before treatment is planned.

Hysteroscopy

Hysteroscopy helps to detect the exact site and size of a submucus fibromyoma.

D and C

Dilatation and curettage should be performed in a case with irregular vaginal bleeding and endometrial biopsy is a must to exclude endometrial carcinoma before treatment is planned.

Differential Diagnosis

The following condition should be considered:

- Full bladder
- Pregnancy
- Ovarian tumor
- Adenomyosis
- Tubo-ovarian mass.

chapter 27

Abnormalities of Urinary System

Urinary system is closely related to the genital system. Several gynecological conditions cause urinary problem. Some patient comes to gynecologist with urinary symptoms alone. The common urinary problems are dealt with here.

❐ FREQUENCY OF MICTURATION

Frequency of micturation is a common complaint. The important cause is urinary tract infection. Usually some predisposing factors play major role to cause urinary tract infection. The women should be asked if the urinary complaints occurred following child birth or abortion or any gynecological operation. Irradiation of pelvis for treatment of gynecological malignancy is another factor favoring urinary infection. Incomplete voiding leads to accumulation of residual urine and invites infection easily as in cystocele or following Wertheim hysterectomy where denervation of urinary bladder is common sequence, resulting in atonic bladder. Catheterization for any reason increases the risk of urinary infection. A post-menopausal woman may complain of burning urination without urinary infection.

❐ SYMPTOMS

Common complaint is frequency of micturation often associated with burning during urination. Cystitis may cause pain in the suprapubic area. Low grade temperature is usual but in severe infection there may be high rise of temperature with chill and rigor. On palpation tenderness is elicited in the suprapubic region.

Urine is cloudy and microscopic examination shows plenty of pus cells under high power field. In severe cases there may be blood in urine. Urine should be sent for culture and sensitivity test.

❐ URINARY INCONTINENCE

Urinary incontinence may be a symptom of some gynecological abnormality or a condition by itself. General and gynecological examination should be performed in every patient with incontinence. Pelvic examination is of primary importance. Presence of vaginal discharge which may mimic incontinence should be excluded first. Urethral atrophy during menopause may predispose urinary incontinence.

Another important cause is relaxation of pelvic support resulting in cystocele, urethrocele, uterine descent and rectocele. Bimanual examination is necessary to exclude any intra-abdominal pathology. Rectal examination is done for pelvic pathology and to detect impaction of fecal material.

Urinary incontinence are of different varities as – true incontinence, stress incontinence, urge incontinence and overflow incontinence.

True Incontinence

It is mainly due to vesicovaginal fistula. It is a communication between the urinary bladder and the vagina. Vesicovaginal fistula is the most common variety of genitourinary fistula. Other varities are ureterovaginal fistula when ureter opens in vagina and urethrovaginal fistula.

The most common cause of vesicovaginal fistula (VVF) is obstetric injury following obstructed labor, leading to avascular necrosis of the bladder wall and the anterior vaginal wall. VVF may follow some obstetric operation, such as craniotomy, decapitation, difficult forceps delivery, caesarean section and cesarean hysterectomy. Fistula may also occur following gynecological operation such as pelvic floor repair, abdominal or vaginal hysterectomy and Wertheim hysterectomy.

History

Patient's first complaint is continuous dribbling of urine per vagina. Dribbling usually follows after few days of difficult delivery. But in operative fistula dribbling or wetting of bed follows immediately after the operation.

On Examination

There is nothing significant on abdominal examination. On vaginal examination patient is found to be wet with typical urinous smell. Vulval and perineal skin shows marks of excoriation owing to chronic irritation of the area by urine.

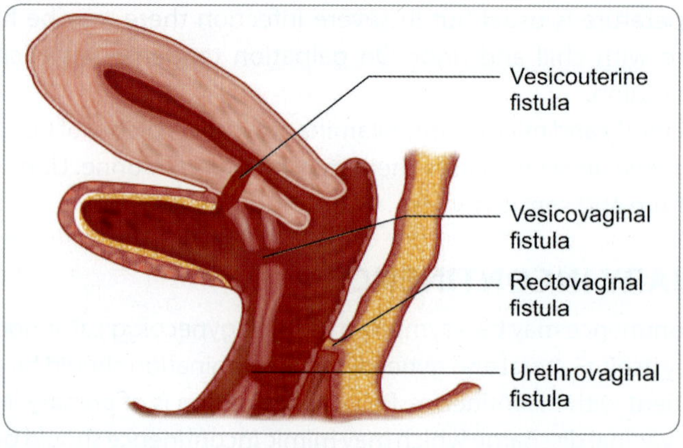

Fig. 1: Different types of urogenital fistula

Speculum examination is an important step as all details of the fistula are obtained. If fistula is present its position, number, size and presence of fibrosis are determined. Patient should be in lithotomy position and a Sim's vaginal speculum is inserted. A big fistula is easily seen as the bladder wall, red in color, protrudes through the fistulous opening. In case of a small fistula a probe is introduced through the urethral meatus and the tip projects through the fistula. Then the size of the fistula and presence of scar tissue around the fistula are assessed. Next is to search for presence of additional fistula.

Dye Test

If the fistula is very small and cannot be visualized, dye test is done. Methylene blue solution is introduced inside the bladder by a rubber catheter. Leakage of dye on the anterior vaginal wall is diagnostic of VVF.

Alternatively, vagina is packed with dry swab. Bladder is filled with about 150 mL of methylene blue solution and the patient is asked to walk for a while. Then putting her again in lithotomy position the swab is taken out and inspected for coloration of the dye. Presence of dye on the swab indicates presence of fistula. If the upper part of the swab is wet but not stained with dye it indicates presence of ureterovaginal fistula.

Bimanual examination is performed to determine the condition of the cervix, the uterus and adnexa. Rectal examination is required specially for detection of rectovaginal fistula which is often present with VVF.

Special procedures required in cases of urinary incontinence are cystoscopy and intravenous pyelography. Cystoscopy is done to determine the position of the fistula in relation to the ureteric openings.

Intravenous pyelography may be needed in certain cases to determine the condition of kidneys and ureters.

To obtain urine sample for culture and sensitivity test the fistulous opening is blocked by passing a Foley catheter through the fistulous opening. The bulb is inflated and gently pulled down to block the opening. Urine sample is collected through a urethral catheter.

Stress Urinary Incontinence

Stress urinary incontinence is the transurethral leakage of urine when intra-abdominal pressure increases as in during coughing, sneezing, etc. Increase of intra-abdominal pressure raises the intravesical pressure to a higher level than the urethral closure pressure can withstand and there occurs leakage of urine. This is true stress incontinence. Detrusor instability may be another cause of stress incontinence.

Patient complains of leakage of urine when intra-abdominal pressure is increased. On examination leakage of urine can be demonstrated when the patient is asked to cough. There may be laxity of anterior vaginal wall also.

Urge Incontinence

Urine leaks involuntarily when there is urgent desire to void. Patient may not be able to reach the toilet even. This is due to bladder irritability. It is usually associated with frequency of micturation, dysuria or stress incontinence.

Overflow Incontinence

There is continuous or intermittent leakage of urine due to over-distention of the urinary bladder. This is commonly a result of neurologic disorder or partial mechanical obstruction to urine flow.

Sophisticated test for urodynamic studies are needed for accurate diagnosis of different types of urinary incontinence.

chapter

28 Pruritus Vulvae

Pruritus vulvae is a symptom of several underlying conditions starting from simple infection to malignancy. It is a distressing condition for a woman who desires to get prompt relief. As such a careful attention and thorough examination is needed.

Among the gynecological conditions trichomonas vaginitis and monilial vulvovaginitis are common to cause intense pruritus. Other local fungal infection and even sometimes pediculosis can cause itching in vulva and perineum. Continuous dribbling of urine in cases of urinary incontinence may cause pruritus. Similarly chronic vaginal discharge being irritating to vulval skin may lead to pruritus.

Vulval dystrophy is another cause of intense vulval pruritus. Metabolic disorders such as diabetes mellitus, chronic liver disease and uremia also cause pruritus vulvae. It may be one of the leading symptoms of diabetes mellitus. Dermatological conditions affecting other parts of the body may cause itching over vulval skin also. Allergy to some food, drugs, linen and napkin used during menstruation may cause pruritus in vulval and perineal region.

Some cases are related to macrocyctic anemia, deficiency of riboflavin, vitamin B_{12} and achlorhydria, etc. In very few cases no cause can be detected. These may be due to some psychological factors. But before labeling it as a sequel of psychological condition other factors leading to pruritus must be excluded.

Vulval dystrophy is a broad term including hyperplastic dystrophy, lichen sclerosus and mixed dystrophy. Hyperplastic dystrophy is commonly seen in post menopausal women, though it may be present in women of reproductive age group also. Formerly this condition was termed as leukoplakia. Vulval skin is thickened and hyperkeratotic. The color of the skin may range from light red to white. Hyperplastic dystrophy may be with cellular atypia which is premalignant. Common symptom is pruritus. Biopsy of effected area is necessary to exclude malignancy.

❑ DERMATOLOGICAL CONDITIONS

Lichen Sclerosus

It is a common white lesion of vulva. This condition is also predominantly seen in post menopausal women. The lesion is flat, pink or white in color with fissures and signs of excoriation. Vulva is atrophic, labia majora is thin and there may be phymosis of prepuce. Pruritus is the common symptom. Patient may complain of dyspareunia. Biopsy is essential.

Mixed Dystrophy

This variety consists of both atrophic and hypertrophic tissue. Symptoms are pruritus, burning and dyspareunia. Biopsy from different areas is needed to exclude cellular atypia or carcinoma.

Detail history taking is essential, keeping in mind the varieties of conditions leading to pruritus vulvae. Duration of pruritus, intensity and presence of vaginal discharge should be enquired. Enquiry should also be made about dribbling of urine and presence of any dermatological conditions in the body. Medical history of diabetes mellitus chronic liver disease and kidney disease should be taken. Allergy to any food material, drug or to sanitary napkin is important to note.

On physical examination of the patient presence of any dermatological lesion should be noted. Attention is needed to exclude any sign of metabolic diseases and of deficiency state. On gynecological examination the condition of the vulva, extent of the lesion, its color and presence of fissures and ulcers on the effected area should be noted. Vaginal examination is done for signs of vaginitis. Cervix should be examined by introducing a speculum. Speculum examination may be difficult in cases of vulval dystrophy.

Complete blood and urine examination should be done to find out any abnormality in relation to the metabolic disorders and the deficiency state. In cases of vulval dystrophy biopsy is necessary.

chapter

29 Carcinoma Vulva

Carcinoma vulva is an uncommon condition. Its etiology is not clear. Older women in their post-menopausal age particularly with long history of vulvitis and pruritus are at higher risk of developing carcinoma vulva. The patients usually give a long history of pruritus vulvae prior to diagnosis of carcinoma. Its relation with vulval dystrophy is not well-established. But there are reports of carcinoma developing on patches of hyperplastic dystrophy or leukoplakia. Carcinoma vulva may be associated with carcinoma of other parts of lower genital tract, such as carcinoma cervix and carcinoma vagina. Presence of human papilloma virus DNA have been reported in patients with vulval carcinoma. Syphilis and other venereal diseases may predispose to this condition.

❒ SYMPTOMS

The common complaints of the patient is swelling over vulva. Patient may give history of vaginal discharge or bleeding. Difficulty in passing urine may be a complaint when urethral meatus or clitoris is involved. Pruritus for a long period of time is a common complaint.

❒ ON EXAMINATION

The commonest site of carcinoma vulva is the labia majora. Usually anterior part of vulva is commonly the site of origin. In few cases labia minora, clitoris or perineum may be the primary site. Multifocal origin of primary lesion is rare.

Usually lesions are ulcerative, raised and leukoplakic. The other variety is nonulcerative. Nonulcerative lesion is flat and indurated. A thorough pelvic examination is needed. On speculum examination the cervix and vaginal walls should be inspected. Pap smear should be taken from cervix. If needed colposcopic-guided biopsy of cervix and vagina should be taken.

Vulva has rich lymphatic supply and lymph gland metastasis is very common. During examination of the patient groin should be palpated to detect enlarged lymph glands.

❐ STAGING

Clinical staging of carcinoma vulva is based on FIGO, 1995, classification. Another staging procedure is TNM classification. Here T stands for the tumor itself, N for lymph node involvement and M for distant metastasis; another method is surgical staging.

Clinical Staging Based on FIGO (1995)

Stage 0

Carcinoma in situ, intraepithelial carcinoma (VIN 3).

Stage 1

Tumor confined to the vulva and/or perineum – 2 cm or less in greatest dimension. Nodes are not palpable.

A. stromal invasion no greater than 1 mm
B. stromal invasion greater than 1 mm.

Stage 2

Tumor confined to the vulva and/or perineum – more than 2 cm in greatest dimension. Nodes are not palpable.

Stage 3

Tumor of any size with:

A. Adjacent spread to the lower urethra and/or the vagina or the anus and/or
B. Unilateral regional node metastasis.

Stage 4

Tumor invades any of the following:

A. Upper urethra, bladder mucosa, rectal mucosa, pelvic bone and/or bilateral regional node metastasis
B. Any distant metastasis including pelvic lymph nodes.

chapter

30 Carcinoma Cervix

❒ PREINVASIVE CARCINOMA OF CERVIX

Cervical intraepithelial neoplasia (CIN) is the preinvasive stage of carcinoma cervix marked by abnormal cellular pattern. To have a better understanding of this microscopic lesion the normal cellular pattern is discussed first.

The cervical canal is lined by mucous membrane thrown into folds. Mucous membrane is lined by a single layer of tall columnar epithelium with basal nucleus. These columnar cells at the top of the folds are ciliated. Clusters of reserve cells are there below the columnar epithelium. Glands are of compound recemose type lined by tall columnar epithelium.

Vaginal portion of the cervix is covered with squamous epithelium and extends upto the external os. The squamous epithelium covering the vagina and exocervix is described in four layers:

Basal layer: It is a single layer of immature cells. Nucleus is large and the cells have small amount of cytoplasm.

Parabasal layer: It has 2–4 layers of immature cells with mitotic figures.

Intermediate layer: It is many layered, cell are polyhydral with large amount of cytoplasm.

Superficial layer: It has many layers of flattened calls with small uniform nucleus, cytoplasm is filled with glycogen. Nucleus of the cells of the more superficial layers are piknotic. These cells exfoliate.

The point at which the endocervical, columnar epithelium and the squamous epithelium of endocervix meet is called squamo columnar junction (SCJ). Squamo columnar junction is a dynamic one. It changes its position in different phases of life, as in puberty, pregnancy and menopause, according to hormonal changes. From neonatal period to menarche SCJ is located at the exocervix. Before menarche there is production of estrogen. Estrogen causes accumulation of glycogen in the vaginal epithelium and lactobacilli acting on glycogen produce lactic acid. Lactic acid makes the vaginal pH acidic, which stimulates the reserve cells to undergo metaplasia. Metaplasia advances to SCJ inwards towards the external os. Now this new SCJ becomes the active SCJ.

The area between the original SCJ and the new SCJ is called transformation zone (TZ). Following menopause SCJ moves further inwards into the cervical canal.

Cervical intraepithelial neoplasia (CIN) is a preinvasive stage of carcinoma cervix. Various terminology was used to describe this phase of evolution of carcinoma cervix. Previously the term dysplasia followed by carcinoma in situ was used to describe the same process. Dysplasia was classified as mild, moderate and severe and then carcinoma in situ. The term CIN has gradually replaced the term dysplasia.

The diagnostic criteria for CIN are cellular immaturity, abnormal cellular organization and nuclear abnormalities.

CIN and dysplasia depends on the depth of involvement of the epithelial layers.

❐ DEGREE OF DYSPLASIA/CIN

Dysplasia	CIN	Depth of involvement
Mild	CIN I	Basal one-third
Moderate	CIN II	Basal two-thirds
Severe	CIN III	Whole thickness
Ca in situ	–	Whole thickness

Bethesda Classification

The Bethesda system classifies the cytological abnormality as atypical squamous cells of undetermined significance (ASCUS), low-grade squamous intraepithelial lesions (LSIL) and high-grade squamous intraepithelial lesion (HSIL).

Oncogenic Irritants

It is believed that oncogenic irritants are introduced through sexual intercourse. As such these include sperm, seminal fluid histone, human papilloma virus (HPV) and herpes simplex virus-2 (HSV–2). Of these two HPV is more important as an irritant.

❐ HISTORY

Patients are Usually Asymptomatic

On clinical examination also there is no specific findings. Some patient may have erosion of cervix. Diagnosis is made by cytological study and biopsy.

Cytological Examination

Cytological study of the cervical scraping and stained by Papanicolaou technique is the standard procedure for cytological screening. Some cytologists may simply report as normal or abnormal smear without attempting in grading the abnormality. Others, however, may indicate as normal, inflammatory or CIN or dysplasia. Doubtful or inconclusive smear indicates repeat smear.

Visualization of Cervix After Application of Acetic Acid

Appearance of white lesion (acetowhite) indicates colposcopy-guided biopsy.

Colposcopy

Colposcope is a device to visualize the cervix, vagina and vulva. Through colposcope an abnormal area of cervical epitheleum can be identified and it becomes easy to select the site for biopsy.
Abnormal colposcopic findings are:

Leukoplakia

Leukoplakia is due to deposition of a layer of kerotin on the surface epithelium. Keratin production on vaginal and cervical epithelium is abnormal. It may be due to HPV infection, keratinizing carcinoma, chronic trauma and radiotherapy. In presence of keratin layer visualization of the underlying epithelium is not possible during colposcopic examination, hence biopsy of the site is indicated.

Punctation

When dilated capillaries terminate on the surface, it appears as a collection of dots. Presence of punctation over an acetowhite epithelium indicates abnormality.

Mosaic

Terminal capillaries encircling roughly circular or polygonal-shaped block of epithelium is called mosaic.

Atypical Vascular Pattern

Vessels of irregular diameter, looped vessels, branching vessels and reticular vessels are an indication of invasive carcinoma.

Irregular surface and ulceration are also abnormal findings.

Cervicograhy

Cervicography is photography of cervix. Cervix is treated with 5% acetic acid and photographs are taken. Films are examined by expert colposcopist. Results of Pap smear, colposcopy and cervicography are correlated and diagnosis is established.

HPV Testing

Koilocytosis is the term given to the cells effected by HPV. These cells are enlarged, nucleus is large with perinuclear halo, irregular and hyperchromatic. There are different types of HP viruses. Of these type 16, 18, 31 and 58 are having more oncogenic potentiality. For detection of HPV DNA different techniques are used as polymerase chain reaction (PCR), southern blot or hybrid culture.

Biopsy

Biopsy should be taken under colposcopic guidance. From endocervix biopsy is taken by a curette and from suspicions area of cervix.

Where colposcope is not available cervix is smeared with 0.3% Schiller's solution or 5% lugols Iodine. Suspicious areas remain unstained and biopsy is taken from that area.

❒ INVASIVE CARCINOMA CERVIX

Carcinoma cervix is a common malignant condition in female genital tract.

Age: Carcinoma cervix has a wide range of age distribution. It is rarely seen in a woman of 20 years and in a woman above 65 years of age. It is commonly seen in the age group of 45–55 years.

❒ SYMPTOMS

The earliest symptom is bleeding per vagina. Bleeding is irregular and of varying amount. Menstruating women usually complain of irregular period or intermenstrual bleeding. In post-menopausal period the woman becomes worried with the episode of bleeding and reports early. Sometimes patient may complain of post-coital bleeding. As the disease progresses bleeding becomes frequent or almost continuous and bleeding may be heavy. The next symptom is vaginal discharge. Initially discharge is thin and foul smelling. Later on it becomes copious and very foul smelling.

Development of pain indicates extension of the disease beyond cervix. Pain may be felt over the back and over the sacrum also. It indicates extension along the utero-sacral ligament. Patients may complain of lower abdominal pain.

❒ ON EXAMINATION

In advanced stage of the disease the patient may be anemic, with ill health, and cachexia may be marked.

Vaginal Examination

On speculum examination in an early case of carcinoma, a nodule or an ulcerated area, which look like erosion, is seen in portio vaginalis. The area bleeds easily when touched with a cotton swab or with the forceps.

In advanced case the lesion looks like a friable mass of cauliflower like growth. Later on it looks like a pedunculated growth filling almost whole of the upper vagina. In other case the lesion looks like an ulcer, which is deep crater like, indurated with raised edge. There is watery, blood stained discharge from the growth or there may be frank bleeding. The discharge is very foul smelling. There may be extension of the lesion.

On palpation a cauliflower type of growth is felt, friable with indurated base. In ulcerative type there is induration and even it may be hard. In early stage endocervical carcinoma may not have any symptom or signs. In later stage of the disease cervix is enlarged, hard and becomes barrel-shaped. When the mass slough a deep excavated lesion is formed and becomes indurated and hard on palpation. In early stage the uterus may be mobile but in advanced stage of the disease mobility is restricted. Palpation of fornices reveals induration in advanced cases, urinary bladder base may also be indurated.

On rectal examination involvement of parametrium is assessed. Depending on the stage of the disease findings vary. In early case there may not be any involvement, whereas in advanced cases parametrial involvement may be there upto the pelvic wall. Involvement of the rectal wall is also assessed in rectal examination.

After history and clinical examination laboratory examination is carried out for confirmation of diagnosis. Confirmation of diagnosis is done by biopsy of the lesion.

❒ DIFFERENTIAL DIAGNOSIS

The following conditions may create confusion and need to be differentiated.

Fibroid Polyp

Fibroid polyp when infected and sloughed may be confused with carcinoma of cervix. On digital examination a fibroid polyp coming out through the external os reveals the origin of the polyp and that it has not originated from the cervix. It is firm on palpation and bleeds but not like a malignant growth.

Cervical Erosion

Usually cervical erosion does not create confusion. The surface of an erosion is velvety. It may have slight oozing but does not bleed heavily like carcinoma cervix.

Tubercular Ulceration

Tubercular ulceration of cervix is soft but not friable. Margins are undermined. Cervical biopsy is needed for confirmation of diagnosis.

Mucus Polyp

Cervical mucus polyp is small, pea shaped, red and pedunculated, protrudes from the cervical canal.

Syphilitic Ulcer

Punched out ulcer with indurated base, smear from the ulcer may demonstrate spirochetes. Biopsy confirms diagnosis.

❒ INVESTIGATIONS

- Routine blood examination is carried out.
- Special investigations are required in selected cases.
- Colposcopy in early cases of carcinoma cervix.
- Cystoscopy to determine involvement of bladder base.
- Intravenous pyelography to evaluate the condition of kidneys and the ureters.
- Proctoscopy and Barium enema may be needed in suspected cases of bowel involvment.
- Chest X-ray is needed to exclude lung metastasis. CT scan and MRI are of special help to assess the extent of the disease, particularly lymph node metastasis.

❒ STAGING

Staging of carcinoma cervix is essential before formulation of mode of treatment. Staging of cervical carcinoma is basically clinical. For staging physical examination of pelvis should be carried out under anesthesia. Help of routine ancillary examination findings such as chest X-ray, colposcopy are taken into account.

Staging of Invasive Carcinoma of cervix

FIGO,1955

Stage I: Carcinoma strictly confined to the cervix (extension to the corpus should be disregarded).

Stage Ia: Preclinical carcinoma of the cervix, that is those diagnosed only by microscopy and not clinically.

Stage Ia_1: Minimal microscopically evident stromal invasion, not exceeding 3 mm.

Stage Ia_2: Microscopically measured invasion greater than 3 mm and not greater than 5 mm and wider than 7 mm (Depth of invasion should not be more than 5 mm taken from the base of the epithelium, either surface or glandular, from which it originates and a second dimension, the horizontal spread must not exceed 7 mm). Larger lesions should be staged as Ib.

Stage Ib: Lesions of greater dimensions than stage Ia_2 whether seen clinically or not. Vascular space involvment should not alter the staging but should be specially recorded so as to determine whether it should affect treatment decisions in the future.

Stage $1b_1$: Lesion not exceeding 4 cm in size.

Stage $1b_2$: Lesion exceeds 4 cm in size

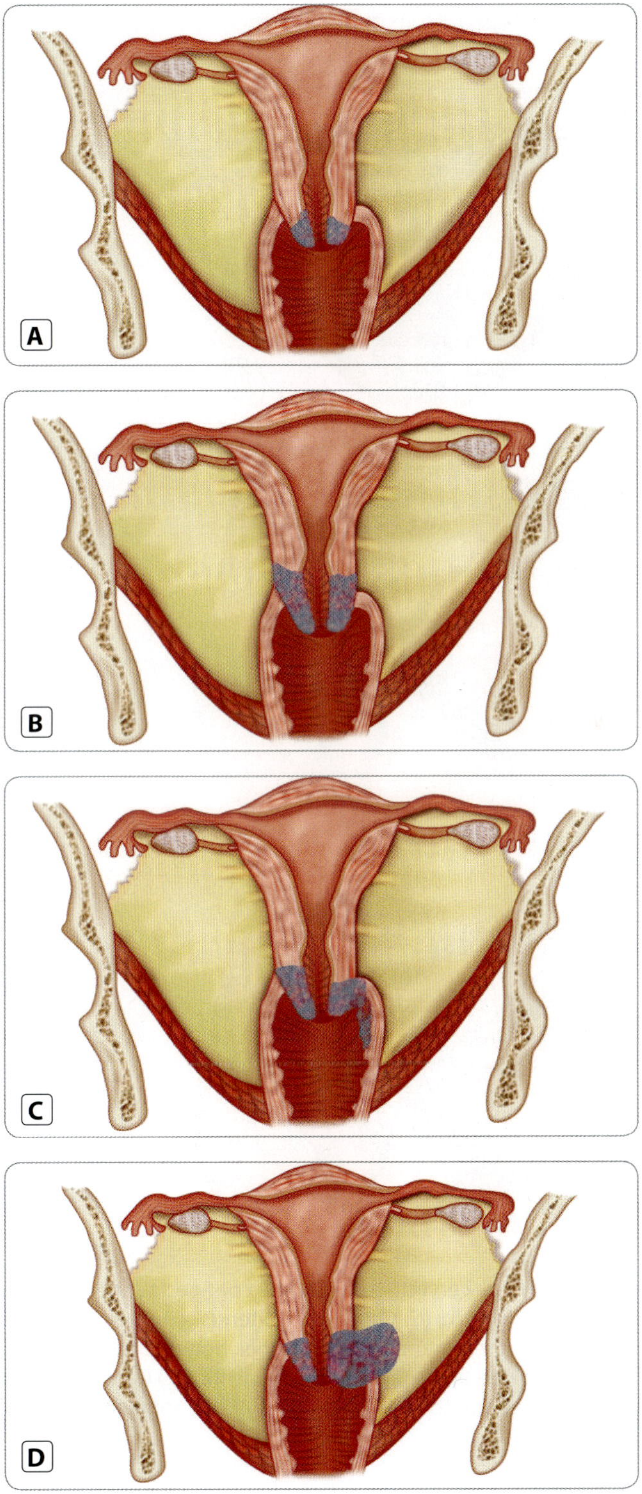

Figures Contd...

Figures Contd...

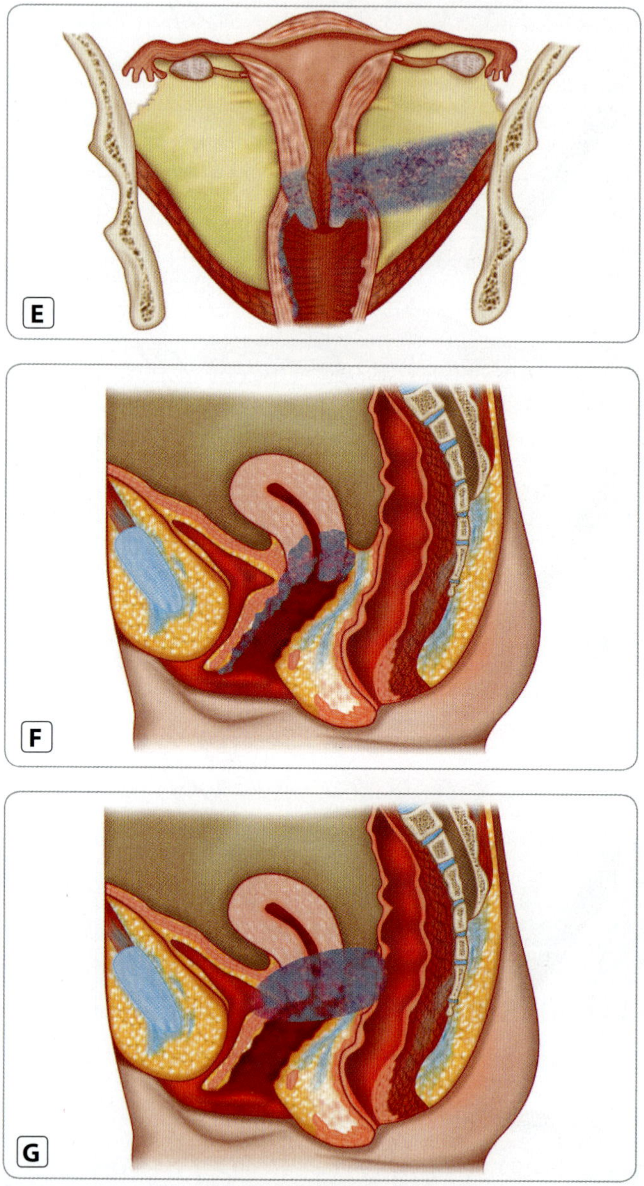

Figs 1A to G: Staging of carcinoma cervix: (A) Carcinoma confined to the cervix – stage Ib; (B) "Barrel shaped" cervix – stage Ib; (C) Carcinoma extends to upper vagina – stage IIa; (D) Carcinoma extends into the parametrium but does not extend to pelvic wall – stage IIb; (E) Parametrium involved upto pelvic wall – stage IIIb; (F) Carcinoma involves anterior vaginal wall upto lower one third – stage IIIa; (G) Carcinoma involves bladder base and rectum – stage IV

Stage II: The carcinoma extends beyond the cervix but has not extend to the pelvic wall. The carcinoma involves the vagina, but not the lower-third.

Stage IIa: No obvious parametrial involvement.

Stage IIb: Obvious parametrial involvement.

Stage III: The carcinoma has extended to the pelvic wall. On rectal examination, there is no cancer-free space between the tumor and the pelvic wall. The tumor involves the lower third of the vagina. All cases with hydronephrosis or non-functioning kidney are included.

Stage IIIa: No extension to the pelvic wall but to the lower-third of vagina.

Stage IIIb: Extension onto the pelvic wall and/or hydronephrosis or non-functioning kidney.

Stage IV: The carcinoma has extended beyond the true pelvis or has clinically involved the mucosa of the bladder or rectum.

A bullous edema as such does not permit a case to be alloted to Stage IV.

Stage IVa: Spread of growth to adjacent organs.

Stage IVb: Spread to distant organs.

chapter

31 Examination of a Patient with Acute Abdomen

Abdominal pain is a common symptom in obstetrics and gynecology. Acute pain is usually sudden and intense in nature or may develop within a few hours. Acute abdomen demands immediate attention of the doctor on duty and urgent treatment. Delay in diagnosis and appropriate management leads to increase mortality and morbidity.

Character of pain differs. Colicky pain is sharp gripping pain comes on suddenly and disappears to reappear again. It comes intermittently. It is often associated with obstruction of a hollow viscous like intestine, ureter or the uterus. Pain may be slow and agonizing usually seen with torsion, constant burning pain in characteristic of peritonitis and throbbing pain is commonly seen with acute inflammation.

❐ ACUTE ABDOMEN DURING PREGNANCY

Changes During Pregnancy

The enlarging pregnant uterus and the changed hormonal status bring about some changes in anatomy and physiology of some of the pelvic organs, that may create confusion in ascertaining the exact origin of pain. During pregnancy the enlarging uterus becomes an abdominal organ by 12 weeks of gestation. The enlarged uterus compresses some public viscera and displaces some. The vermiform appendix is displaced upwards making diagnosis of acute appendicitis difficult. Due to increased level of circulating progesterone esophageal sphincter pressure is lowered and gastric emptying time is delayed. The former can lead to heart burn and esophageal reflux and the later leads to nausea and vomiting.

In urologic system also increased progesterone concentration dilates the ureter through its effect on the smooth muscles of the ureters. Secondly, the enlarging uterus presses over the ureter leading to its dilatation proximal to the level of compression. This effect is more prominent on the right side because of the slight tilting of the uterus towards the right side. Ureteric dilatation results in urinary stasis inviting infection. Urinary infection is more common in primigravida women around 20 weeks of gestation.

Causes of Acute Abdomen During Pregnancy – Appendicitis

The incidence of acute appendicitis during pregnancy is found to be 1 in 1500 pregnancies. The presenting symptoms are acute pain over right lower quadrant of abdomen, usually associated with anorexia, nausea, vomiting and slight rise of temperature. Later on, fever may be high. Initially pain starts around the umbilicus and gradually settles down in the right iliac fossa as in non-pregnant state. Local signs like rebound tenderness and muscle guard are delayed to appear due to the presence of the gravid uterus, which may delay the diagnosis of acute appendicitis.

Gallbladder Disease

Acute cholecystitis without biliary sludge or gallstone, during pregnancy is not uncommon. Gallstone formation is predisposed by pregnancy. It is suggested that increased circulation of sex steroids during pregnancy delays gallbladder emptying and favors gallstone formation.

In acute condition the patient presents with pain in right upper quadrant of abdomen, nausea, vomiting and may be associated with fever. On examination along with tachycardia there is tenderness over the right upper quadrant of abdomen. Abdominal ultrasonography may reveal gallstone or biliary sludge with signs of inflammation.

Other gastrointestinal causes of acute abdomen are intestinal obstruction, pancreatitis, etc.

❒ RENAL CAUSES

A gravid woman with kidney stone may present with severe pains in loins, nausea, vomiting and may be accompanied by hematuria. In ureteric colic due to ureteric obstruction by calculus may present with severe excruciating pain on one side of the abdomen, particularly on back and/or in the flanks. For diagnosis of renal calculus abdominal ultrasonography may not be of much help as the visualization of kidneys and ureters is not adequate due to the presence of the enlarged gravid uterus. Help of urologist should be sought for proper management of the patient.

Another common condition relating to the urinary system is acute urinary infection. In acute infection there is acute pain over the suprapubic region, may be associated with loin pain, dysuria and fever. Nausea and vomiting are usually present. On examination there is tachycardia, tenderness over the suprapubic region and over the loin. Examination of urine shows plenty of pus cells and bacteria. Culture and sensitivity test of urine reveals the causative organism.

❒ OBSTETRICAL CAUSES

Abortion: Abortion or miscarriage is a common complication of early pregnancy. About 10–15 per cent of diagnosed pregnancy ends in abortion. In threatened and missed abortion the woman may feel mild pain in suprapubic region and may be associated with slight vaginal bleeding. But in inevitable abortion the product of conception is expelled partly or completely.

In this process the uterus contracts to open the closed cervix and to expel the product of conception. The woman feels sharp, gripping pain over the suprapubic region. Sometimes the pain is very severe accompanied by vaginal bleeding. Bleeding may be very severe necessitating immediate surgical removal of the product of conception.

On examination of the woman there is tachycardia, blood pressure may vary depending on the amount of blood loss. Suprapubic area may be tender. On vaginal examination uterus is found to be enlarged, cervix is open and in incomplete abortion product of conception may be felt inside the cervical canal.

Disturbed Ectopic Pregnancy

In ectopic pregnancy the pregnancy sac is implanted in a site other than the uterine cavity. The commonest site is the fallopian tubes. Usually diagnosis of disturbed ectopic pregnancy is not difficult, but sometimes it may be problematic, particularly in pregnancy with an intact gestational sac.

Patient gives history of short period of amenorrhea followed by pain in lower abdomen. There may be slight bleeding per vaginum. Usually onset of pain is associated with fainting attack of short duration. Referred pain to the right shoulder may develop as a result of irritation of the diaphragm by blood traversing through right paracolic gutter. Accumulation of blood and blood clot in the pouch of Douglas may lead to urge to defecate and accumulation of blood in utero-vesical pouch may cause frequency of micturation.

On examination tachycardia and low blood pressure are common. Blood pressure depends on the amount of bleeding inside the abdomen. Even if blood pressure is within normal limit tachycardia is a must with pallor. Again the degree of pallor depends on the amount of blood loss. On abdominal examination whole abdomen, particularly the lower abdomen is very tender with muscle guard. There may be slight distention of the abdomen with reduced peristaltic sound. There is evidence of fluid in the flanks. Vaginal examination is painful. Pelvis is tender and movement of the cervix increases tenderness. A

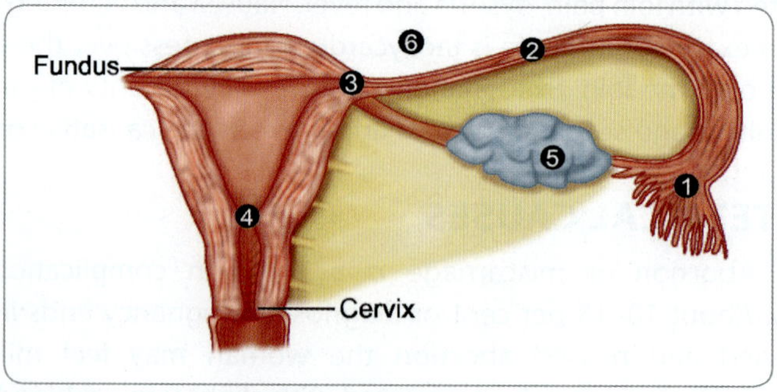

Fig. 1: Different sites of ectopic pregnancy. 1–Fimbrial; 2– Isthemic; 3–Cornual; 4–Cervical; 5–Ovarian

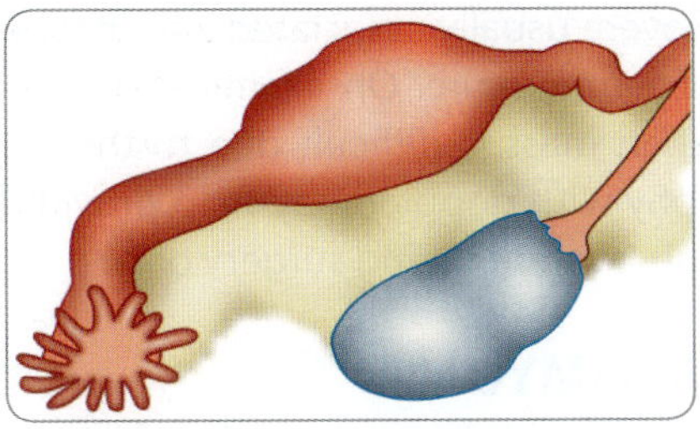

Fig. 2: Unruptured tubal ectopic pregnancy

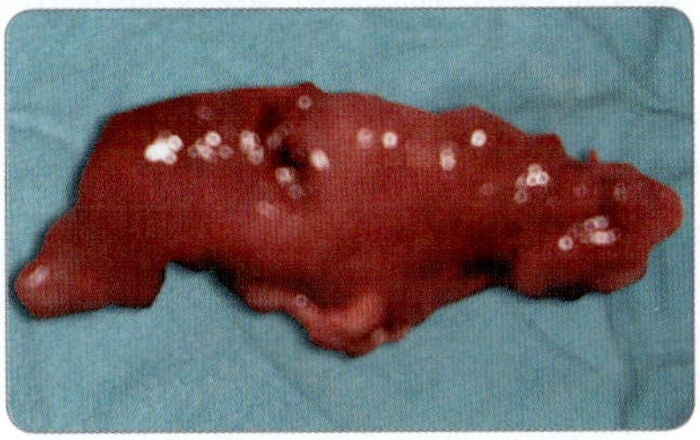

Fig. 3: Unruptured tubal pregnancy, window shows hematoma inside

soft mass fills the pouch of Douglas. It is better to avoid manipulation of the pelvis, so that the clot is not disturbed.

❒ DIAGNOSIS

History: Symptoms and signs are important to focus the attention of the attending doctor towards the diagnosis of ectopic pregnancy. Urine should be examined for pregnancy test which shows positive reaction. Ultrasonographic examination done after rupture of the ectopic pregnancy may show a complex adnexal mass with evidence of free peritoneal fluid. Before rupture of the fallopian tube with ectopic pregnancy it is sometimes very difficult to diagnose even with ultrasonography. A careful correlation of clinical findings, urine test results and ultrasonographic findings is needed to arrive at a diagnosis. Sometimes repeat ultrasound examination is needed.

Ruptured corpus luteum cyst of pregnancy presents with the same picture. Presence of intrauterine gestational sac on ultrasonography helps in differentiating from disturbed ectopic pregnancy.

❒ TORSION OF OVARIAN TUMOR

Torsion of ovarian tumor during pregnancy occurs mostly in mid-pregnancy or in early puerperium. Torsion of the pedicle containing the vascular supply to the ovary leads to ischemia of the ovary and results in acute pain abdomen. Torsion commonly occurs in a benign cystic teratoma of moderate size which is heavier with a long pedicle.

Pain of torsion is severe usually associated with nausea, vomiting and may be with slight rise of temperature. On examination the abdomen is tender. Palpation of the ovarian mass is difficult due to the presence of the gravid uterus. Ultrasonography with doppler may help providing more information. Many a times diagnosis is made during surgery only.

❐ UTERINE FIBROMYOMA

Complications of uterine fibromyoma during pregnancy may present with acute abdomen. During pregnancy size of the fibroid may increase and may undergo red degeneration. Pain in lower abdomen may be associated with nausea, vomiting and slight rise of temperature. On physical examination tenderness is elicited over the region of the tumor. Signs of peritoneal irritation may also be found. There may be leukocytosis, ultrasonography is helpful to detect the fibromyoma.

❐ GYNECOLOGICAL CONDITIONS

Dysmenorrhea

Dysmenorrhea is painful menstruation. Sometimes with severe colicky pain the women becomes incapacitated to do her daily work.

Two types of dysmenorrhea are described – primary and secondary. Primary dysmenorrhea is mainly seen in adolescent girls, pain is colicky in nature. Pain starts usually with onset of menstruation and lasts for about 1–2 days. Often it lasts for few hours only. Pain may be very severe and the woman may remain tossing over the bed.

In primary dysmenorrhea no definite pelvic pathology is found. Secondary dysmenorrhea is usually associated with some gynecological condition. These are chronic pelvic infection, endometriosis, adenomyosis, fibromyoma of uterus, etc. Pain in pelvic infection is felt 4–5 days before onset of menstruation, dull aching in nature, usually confined to the lower abdomen and relieved by onset of menstrual flow. In endometriosis pain starts after onset of menstruation, may be very severe and may last for 3–4 days after cessation of menstrual flow, urination and defecation may aggravate pain. Adenomyosis is almost always associated with severe pain. But in fibromyoma of uterus pain is uncommon. Patient feels pain during periods if the myoma is situated near the cornual end of the uterus or if a fibromyomatous polyp is in the process of expulsion from the uterine cavity. Abdominal and pelvic examination reveal the cause of pain. In some cases ultrasonographic help is necessary.

Complications of Ovarian Tumor

Cystic ovarian neoplasia undergoes some complications leading to acute abdomen. Torsion or rupture of the cyst are common conditions.

Torsion of Ovarian Neoplasm

Torsion is a common complication of cystic neoplasia of ovary. Torsion occurs at the pedicle of the cystic tumor. Torsion leads to ischemia and onset of acute pelvic pain. Benign cystic teratoma commonly undergoes torsion because of its heavy nature with a long pedicle. Symptoms of torsion are same as during pregnancy. On clinical examination a tender lump in lower quadrant of the abdomen can be felt. There is rebound tenderness. Delineation of the cystic mass may be difficult due to presence of tenderness and muscle guard. There may be slight rise of temperature with tachycardia. Ultrasonography of lower abdomen and pelvis confirms the presence of the cystic mass.

Clinical examination and history of presence of a mass in lower abdomen are sufficient for diagnosis.

Rupture of Ovarian Cyst

Benign cystadenoma and benign cystic teratoma of ovary may rupture and may cause acute abdominal pain. Chocolate cyst of ovary also can rupture producing signs and symptoms of acute abdomen. Rarely rupture of corpus luteum cyst may lead to hemoperitoneum and presents a state of acute abdomen. This may mimic the symptoms of ruptured ectopic pregnancy.

Patient presents with acute abdominal pain. On examination tachycardia is present and in case of hemoperitoneum blood pressure may be low. Abdomen is tender with rebound tenderness and distension.

Diagnosis depends on history, clinical findings, complete blood count and ultrasonographic examination of abdomen. To differentiate from disturbed ectopic pregnancy urine for pregnancy test should be done.

Acute Salpingo-oophoritis

Acute salpingo-oophoritis is an acute infection of the fallopian tube, ovary and the surrounding structures. It is almost always bilateral. It may follow abortion or delivery. Usually it is an ascending infection from vagina and cervix. Infection can also occur from sexually transmitted pathogens.

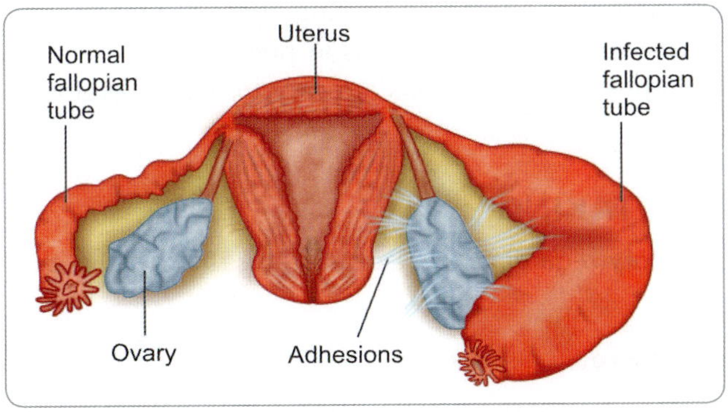

Fig. 4: Pelvic inflammatory disease with hydrosalpinx

Common symptoms are acute lower abdominal pain with rise in temperature and may be associated with nausea, vomiting and vaginal discharge.

On examination lower abdomen is tender with tachycardia and rise of temperature. On vaginal examination fornices are tender, tenderness increases with movement of the cervix. An inflammatory lump may be felt through the fornices. Blood examination reveals leukocytosis. To ascertain the offending pathogen high vaginal swab culture is needed.

❐ ENDOMETRIOSIS

Endometriosis is a condition where ectopic endometrium is present outside the endometrial cavity of the uterus. Pain of endometriosis is usually cyclical and acute pain occurs premenstrually or during menstruation. Rupture of a chocolate cyst also leads to acute abdominal pain.

On examination tenderness is present over suprapubic region. Sometimes tender lump may be felt on either side of midline.

On vaginal examination pelvis is tender and uterus is fixed. Tender nodules can be felt in the uterosacral ligaments. Ultrasonography is helpful in the diagnosis of endometriosis. Laparoscopic examination is needed to confirm the diagnosis.

Urologic Causes

Women with cystitis and pyelonephritis may present with acute abdominal pain. Another common urologic cause is ureteric colic due to ureteric calculus. In this condition pain is sudden, excruciating and colicky in nature. Hematuria is often present. Cystitis is associated with dull aching pain felt mostly in the suprapubic region accompanied by dysuria, hematuria and frequency of micturation.

Urine analysis in a case of urinary tract infection reveals plenty of pus cell and red blood cells.

For ureteric lithiasis ultrasonography or intravenous pyelography is needed to locate the calculus. Urine culture is essential to know the infective organism.

Gastrointestinal tract: Conditions arising from the gastrointestinal tract leading to acute abdomen are same as in pregnancy. The difference is that during the non-pregnant state signs are easy to elicit, therefore, diagnosis is easier.

❐ HISTORY TAKING

A complete history regarding age, social status, food habit, occupation are taken.

Menstrual History

Menstrual history is important in a woman of reproductive age. The cycle, period and flow of menstruation are important. Dysmenorrhea is a condition occuring only during menstruation. Pain of gynecological origin may be related to menstruation.

Personal History

History of life style of the woman should be enquired as it influences the behavior of the woman.

Social Status

The first thing to know is whether the woman is married or unmarried. If married when she was married should be enquired and noted.

Past Obstetric History

Detail past obstetric history is important to correlate pelvic pain with previous abortion or child birth. Some conditions like endometriosis, adenomyosis or uterine fibromyoma are associated with inability to conceive or with abortion.

❒ CHIEF COMPLAINTS

Pain: Everything relating to pain should be enquired. Onset of pain in relation to menstruation or whether the patient feels pain during the intermenstrual period are significant for diagnosis of the cause of pain. Mode of onset of pain whether sudden or gradual, ending in severe pain needs attention. Past history of pain abdomen, if any, and how she got relief should be noted. Exact site of pain and its radiation to back or towards the thighs is enquired. Enquiry should be made about, the character of pain, i.e. whether dull aching, colicky or throbbing which indicates different conditions for cause of pain. Another important point to be asked is relation of pain with micturation, defecation and coitus. Next is how the pain is relieved.

Is pain associated with nausea, vomiting and rise of temperature?

❒ PHYSICAL EXAMINATION

Thorough physical examination is very important to arrive at a provisional diagnosis. As a first step the patient is observed carefully to notice her general appearance and attitude.

In colic the patient may be tossing on the bed or doubled up. In case of intraperitoneal hemorrhage patient is extremely pale with severe pain in abdomen. A patient with peritonitis remains quite as movement increases pain.

Pulse and Blood Pressure

A patient with acute abdominal pain from any cause usually has tachycardia. In intraperitoneal hemorrhage pulse of the patient is a good indicator. In initial stage blood pressure may remain normal but at later stage hypotension is present.

Temperature

In infection like acute appendicitis, severe cystitis temperature may be raised, mild rise of temperature may be present in torsion of ovarian cyst, otherwise rise of temperature is not a common finding.

Pallor

Marked pallor is an important feature of intraperitoneal hemorrhage.

Abdominal Examination

Abdominal examination and vaginal examination should be carried out systematically and findings should be noted. Method of examination is discussed in chapter 8.

Laboratory Test

Patients with acute pain should undergo the following tests to arrive at a definite diagnosis.

Routine blood examination includes hemoglobin concentration, erythrocytic sedimentation rate, total white cell count and differential leukocytic count. Total white cell count is raised in active infection with leukocytosis found in differential leukocytic count.

Urine analysis for protein, glucose and presence of pus cell is helpful.

In doubtful cases urine for pregnancy test is needed.

Urine for culture and sensitivity test should be done to exclude urinary infection.

Pelvic ultrasonography is helpful in the diagnosis of ectopic pregnancy, to confirm the findings of clinical examination in case of adnexal mass. Adenomyosis can be differentiated from uterine fibromyoma.

X-ray of the abdomen is useful in differentiating few gastrointestinal problems. X-ray of abdomen should be avoided during pregnancy.

CT scan, MRI: CT scan and MRI are used to get detail informations of a pelvic mass, retroperitoral mass, abcess and of hemoperitoneum.

❐ LAPAROSCOPY

Diagnostic laparoscopy is very helpful to establish the diagnosis in a doubtful case. Direct visualization of the abdominal viscera helps the physician to examine the nature of a pelvic mass and to ascertain the cause of hemoperitoneum. But in acute condition one should be aware of the relative contraindication like hypovolumic shock, peritonitis, intestinal obstruction, etc.

chapter

32 Investigative Procedures

After history taking and physical examination of the patient few laboratory investigations are needed to arrive at a diagnosis. The relevant findings of history and physical examination are correlated with the findings of the laboratory investigations to arrive at a final diagnosis. In this modern era of advanced and sophisticated biotechnology, numerous investigative procedures are available. Here, only those which are needed at the primary stage and can be performed easily will be discussed in brief. A student should be familiar with these basic investigative procedures.

❒ EXAMINATION OF BLOOD

For examination blood is drawn by venepuncture and collected in sterile vials. According to the type of examination required the vial should contain appropriate anticoagulant in right proportion, to the amount of blood. After putting the blood in vial, the vial should be shaked to prevent clot formation. In the examinations where serum is needed the vials are empty and after putting blood it should not be shaked, so that the clot can form and serum is separated. Then the vial is labelled and sent to laboratory.

❒ INVESTIGATIONS

Routine blood examination includes hemoglobin (Hb) concentration, total leukocytic count (TC), differential leukocytic count (DLC), erythrocyte sedimentation rate (ESR), ABO and Rho grouping.

For determination of glucose concentration in blood random blood sugar, fasting and postprandial blood sugar are done. In suspected cases and in high risk patients oral glucose tolerance test (OGTT), after 75 g of glucose ingestion should be done. Blood is examined every ½ hourly for 2–3 hours of glucose ingestion. In pregnant woman amount of glucose to be taken should be 100 g. Fasting blood glucose is determined after 8–14 hours of fasting (overnight fasting). Another simple test is glucose challenge test (GCT). In this screening test blood glucose concentration is estimated 1 hour after ingestion of 50 g of glucose.

Liver function tests are done in some patients. These tests are not necessary routinely. These include alkaline phosphatase, bilirubin and its fractions, aspartate aminotransferase (AST/SGOT), alanine aminotransferase (ALT/SGPT), total protein and its fractions, etc.

Renal function tests are done as required for pre-operative evaluation and in some pregnant woman also. These include blood urea, urea nitrogen (BUN), serum creatinine and uric acid, etc.

Lipid profile includes total cholesterol level, triglycerides, high-density lipoprotein (HDL), low-density lipoprotein (LDL), etc.

In thyroid profile free thyroxine level and level of thyroid stimulating hormone are estimated.

In certain situation blood coagulation profile is needed. The examinations commonly done are bleeding time, coagulation time, platelet count, prothrombin time, fibrinogen concentration, etc.

Besides those mentioned here there are various other tests which are done as and when the situation demands.

❐ EXAMINATION OF URINE

Urine examination is needed to know the function of the urinary system. Few basic examination can be done by the attending nurse or by the doctor on duty.

Collection of Urine Specimen

Urine should be collected in a wide mouthed dry, clean container. It should be covered, labeled and sent to laboratory.

Type of Urine Specimen

Early Morning Urine Specimen is the Most Concentrated Urine

Random Specimen is Collected at any Time of the Day

Twenty Four Hour Urine Specimen

Urine is collected from morning till next morning. The first morning urine of the first day is not collected. All the urine passed during the first day and night is collected including the first urine of the next morning. Urine should be collected in a wide mouthed clean container. The bottle is sealed, labeled and sent to laboratory.

Mid Stream Urine Collection

The patient is provided with a wide mouthed clean container and instructed to collect the urine during the middle of the act of urination.

Urine Collected Using a Catheter

Urine should be collected in hospital by a doctor or a nurse. Care should be taken to maintain a sterile condition. Hands are washed, dried and sterile gloves are put on. Patient should lie in dorsal position, thighs are kept apart. Labia are separated with the fingers of the left hand. Urethral meatus is cleaned with a sterile cotton swab. A sterile catheter is held by the fingers of the right hand away from the tip and the tip is gently introduced inside the urethra and the urinary bladder. Urine is collected in a sterile container.

Collection of Vaginal Discharge

Specimen of vaginal discharge is taken before internal examination. A posterior vaginal speculum is introduced, without using any lubricant, and specimen is collected by a sterile swab stick. The swab stick is immediately put into a sterile test tube, labeled and sent to laboratory.

The two common organisms causing vaginitis are *trichomonas vaginalis* and *candida albicans*. These organisms can be easily identified in a side laboratory.

Trichomonas Vaginalis

- One drop of discharge is taken on a dry, clean glass slide. Mix with one drop of normal saline.
- Put a cover slip.
- Examine under microscope.

Actively motile trichomonas are seen easily. Culture is rarely indicated. Culture media are Kupferberg's media or Feinberg Whittington media.

Monilia

- Put a drop of discharge on a glass slide
- Put a drop of potassium hydroxide mix
- Cover with a cover slip
- See under microscope, or
- Spread the discharge on a glass slide, dried and stain with methylene blue
- Look under microscope.

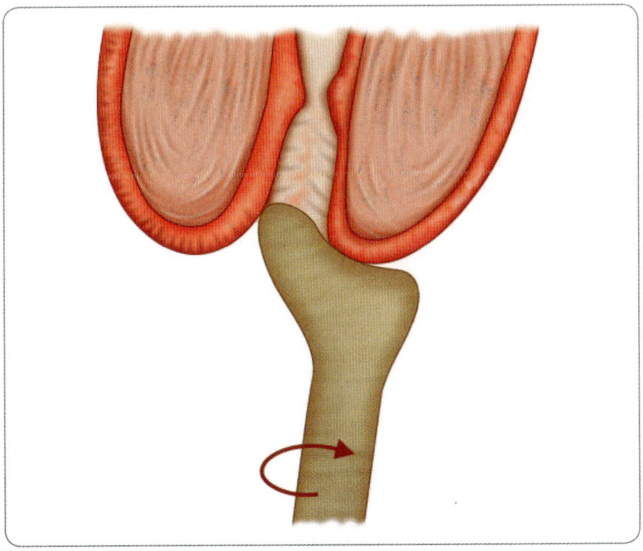

Fig. 1: Taking of cervical smear for pap staining

The mycele of fungus can be seen under microscope. For culture, media are Nickerson's media or Subouraud's media.

Pap Smear

Advice to patient before taking the smear:

- Not to use any vaginal cream or pessary for at least one week
- To abstain from sexual intercourse for 24 hours
- Smear is taken from both the endocervix and exocervix.

Materials

- Cotton tipped swab moist in normal saline or cervical brush
- Ayre's spatula
- Clean glass slide
- Koplin jar or any other suitable container with fixative, 95% ether and alcohol.

Taking Cervical Smear with Ayer's Specula

Procedures:

- Patient is put in dorsal or lithotomy position.
- No lubricant should be used in the speculum.
- Speculum is introduced inside the vagina.
- Put the cotton tipped swab or the brush inside the cervical canal and taking it out spread the sample on a clean glass slide and put the slide immediately inside the Koplin jar containing the fixative.
- Place the spatula against the cervix with the longer protrusion in the cervical canal.
- Rotate the spatula clockwise 360 degree firmly against the cervix.
- Spread the sample on a glass slide.
- Put the slide immediately into fixative.

Care should be taken to avoid air drying before putting the slides into fixative. The smear should be thick and after fixing for 30 minutes the slides can be taken out air-dried and sent for laboratory or can be sent with the jar also, if the laboratory is attached to the clinic.

❐ COLPOSCOPY

Colposcope is an instrument designed to visualize the exocervix. Magnification is about 15 to 40 times.

The procedure should be explained to the patient. It needs no anesthesia.

Procedure

- Patient should be in lithotomy position.
  - Legs are draped with sterile linen
  - Bringing the colposcope in position inspect the vulva and perineum for ulceration or inflammation

- Inserting the speculum, vagina is inspected to detect ulceration or discharge.

- Clean the cervix of discharge and cellular debris using a swab soaked with normal saline.
- Using low power magnification examine the cervix. Identify the columnar epithelium and the original squamocolumnar junction.
- Apply 3% acetic acid with a cotton swab to the cervix and upper vagina, continue examination.
- Acetic acid causes coagulation of the nuclear protein which is high in CIN and the area looks white (acetowhite).
- Look for punctation and mosaic pattern.
- Apply a green filter and examine the cervix, green filter helps in identifying the vessels.
- Perform endocervical curettage under colposcopic vision.
- Perform colposcopically directed biopsy of the cervix when needed.
- Photograph is taken before endometrial biopsy.

❐ CERVICAL BIOPSY

Cervical biopsy is mandatory for diagnosis of cervical carcinoma.

Different types of biopsy are described below:

Punch Biopsy

Punch biopsy is taken as an outpatient procedure without anesthesia. Cervix is exposed introducing a vaginal speculum. Anterior lip of the cervix is held with a volselum. Biopsy is taken from the suspected areas with the help of punch biopsy forceps. It is better to stain the cervix with Schiller's iodine and biopsy is taken from the unstained areas.

Wedge Biopsy

In this procedure a wedge-shaped portion of the cervix is taken for biopsy. Necrotic tissue should be avoided and should include a part of healthy tissue, as an edge of the lesion is the ideal site.

Cervix is exposed introducing a posterior vaginal speculum and lips are held with long Allies forceps. The selected area is cut with a scalpel and the piece of tissue is collected. To stop bleeding suturing may be needed or a vaginal pack is kept.

Cone Biopsy

In this procedure a cone of the cervix is removed. The base of the cone should include the squamocolumnar junction and the apex should be below the internal os. It is performed under general anesthesia.

Hemostatic sutures are applied in the cone margin.

Complications of Cone Biopsy

1. Secondary hemorrhage
2. Cervical stenosis
3. Cervical incompetence leading to mid-trimester abortion, premature labor.

For biopsy tissue obtained should be placed in 10% formalin and send to laboratory. Tissue needed for frozen-section examination must be delivered to the laboratory immediately without fixative.

❒ OTHER DIAGNOSTIC PROCEDURES IN GYNECOLOGY

Other diagnostic procedures in gynecology are invasive in nature and performed in operation theater, preferably under general anesthesia. These are:

Dilatation and Curettage

It is mostly a diagnostic procedure in which endometrium is curetted out and sent to laboratory for histopathological examination. In certain condition it is done for therapeutic purpose also.

In this procedure, in operation theater, the patient is put in lithotomy position. Anesthesia is administered. Patient is asked to evacuate urinary bladder before putting her on operation table. Initially a bimanual examination is done to note the size, shape, direction of the uterus. Then cervix is dilated with cervical dilator followed by uterine curettage.

Diagnostic Indications

- Dysfunctional uterine bleeding
- Any abnormal uterine bleeding
- Infertility
- Suspected endometrial tuberculosis
- Suspected carcinoma endometrium
- Post-menopausal bleeding
- Chorion epithelioma.

Complication

- Injury to cervix
- Uterine perforation
- Infection.

Laparoscopy

Laparoscope is a device to visualize the peritoneal cavity. It is performed in operation theater under general anesthesia. It requires complete preoperative evaluation and preparation of the patient.

Under general anesthesia anterior abdominal wall is perforated and CO_2 gas is introduced to achieve pneumoperitonium. Then the laparoscope fitted with fiber optic light (coldlight) and camera is introduced inside the peritoneal cavity. Pictures are obtained from the TV monitor.

Diagnostic Indications

- In infertility evaluation–tubal pathology, endometriosis, pelvic adhesion, etc. Chromopertubation is done to detect tubal patency.
- To determine the origin and nature of pelvic mass.
- Chronic pelvic pain.
- Acute pelvic pain.
- Amenorrhea (other than in pregnancy).
- Congenital abnormality of uterus.
- For follow-up of pelvic surgery for:
  - Ovarian malignancy
  - Endometriosis
  - Tuboplasty.
- Perforation of uterus.

Hysteroscopy

In this procedure the uterine cavity is visualized.

Indications

- Irregular uterine bleeding
- Post-menopausal bleeding
- Intrauterine adhesion
- Missing IUCD
- Recurrent abortion to detect intrauterine septum and/or intrauterine adhesion.

chapter

33 Radiology and Ultrasonography in Obstetrics and Gynecology

❐ RADIOLOGY

The following radiological examinations are helpful:

- Chest X-ray is needed to exclude secondary metastasis in malignant conditions of pelvis. Chest X-ray is necessary for pre-operative evaluation of a patient.
- Plain picture of abdomen and pelvis helps to locate a lost IUCD. Sometimes a plain picture may reveal a tooth or bony tissue in begin cystic teratoma.

❐ HYSTEROSALPINGOGRAPHY

In this procedure a radio opaque dye is introduced into the uterine cavity, which travels through the fallopian tubes and come out through the fimbrial end of the tubes to the peritoneal cavity. Radiographs are taken which enables to detect any abnormality in the uterine cavity and the fallopian tubes.

It is performed in radiology department. The dye introduced is water-soluble iodine – Diaginol viscus. Water soluble dye is preferred to oil-soluble dye, because:

- It is safe
- Absorption is better
- Negligible peritoneal irritation
- No chance of granuloma formation.

Indications

- In investigation of infertility to detect tubal patency.

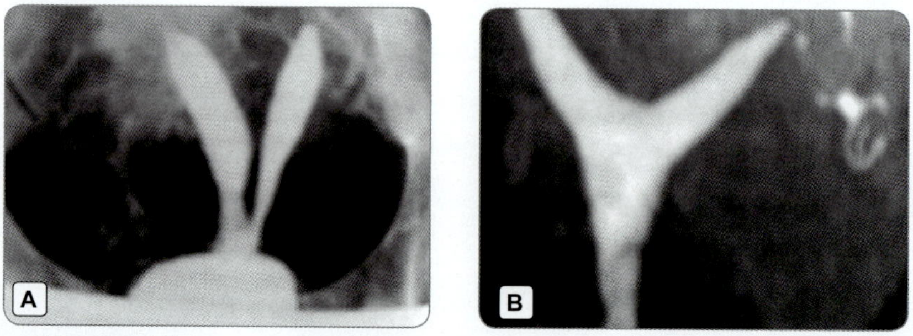

Figs 1A and B: (A) Hysterosalpingography of septate uterus; (B) Hysterosalpingography of bicornuate uterus

- In recurrent abortion to detect uterine abnormality or submucus fibromyoma distorting the uterine cavity.
- For diagnosis of cervical incompetence.
- For diagnosis of uterine Synechie.
- Lost IUCD.

Contraindications

- Pregnancy
- Active vaginal bleeding
- Active pelvic inflammatory disease, vaginal or cervical infection
- Allergic to iodine preparation. In that case other radio opaque dye is to be selected.

The best time to perform the test is 7–10 days after the onset of menstruation.

Procedure

- Bladder should be empty
- Patient in dorsal position
- Vaginal speculum introduced, catch the cervical lip
- Introduce a canula through the cervical canal
- Introduce the dye inside the uterus through the canula
- Remove the speculum and the volselum
- Radiograph is taken under fluroscopic control
- Remove the canula
- Another radiograph is taken after 10–15 minutes
- Tubal patency is evidenced by peritoneal spillage of dye.

Complication

- Pelvic pain from peritoneal irritation
- Vasovagal attack
- Pelvic infection may flare up.

Other radiological procedures include intravenous pyelography and barium enema. These investigations are not always needed in gynecology, but are helpful sometimes for diagnosis or for preoperative evaluation of the patient in certain conditions.

ULTRASONOGRAPHY IN OBSTETRICS AND GYNECOLOGY

Ultrasonography is a unique presentation of modern biotechnology to the physician. The precise diagnosis of different maternal and fetal conditions during pregnancy has undoubtedly improved the pregnancy outcome.

Similarly in the gynecology the precise and accurate diagnosis of pelvic conditions has made the job of the gynecologist in decision making easier and rewarding. Addition of color Doppler has made diagnosis of pelvic mass particularly pelvic malignancy more accurate.

Use of transvaginal ultrasonography has revolutionized the diagnosis and management of early pregnancy complications. In vaginal sonography the transducer is placed near the ovaries. High resolution transvaginal ultrasonography can accurately demonstrate the yolk sac, fetal pole and cardiac activity much earlier than in abdominal ultrasound. Thereby it is possible to differentiate between intact pregnancy from an abnormal pregnancy.

With the help of ultrasonography the doctor can "see" the fetus, its growth, heart beat, body movements, etc. These fetal activities supply some vital informations, regarding well-being of the fetus. On the other hand it has no known risk for the mother and the fetus as well. The increasing use has to some extent reduced the perinatal mortality rate.

Indications of Ultrasonography in Obstetrics

In obstetrics ultrasonography is used in many conditions.

To make it easy to remember, the indications are described trimester-wise.

Indications in first trimester of pregnancy: In day-to-day practice ultrasonography is not used for diagnosis of pregnancy. Immunological examination of urine for detection of β-subunit of human chorionic gonadotropin (hCG) is sufficient for diagnosis of early pregnancy. But in certain situations like pregnancy following rape or in pregnancy following previous recurrent early pregnancy loss, ultrasonographic documentation of

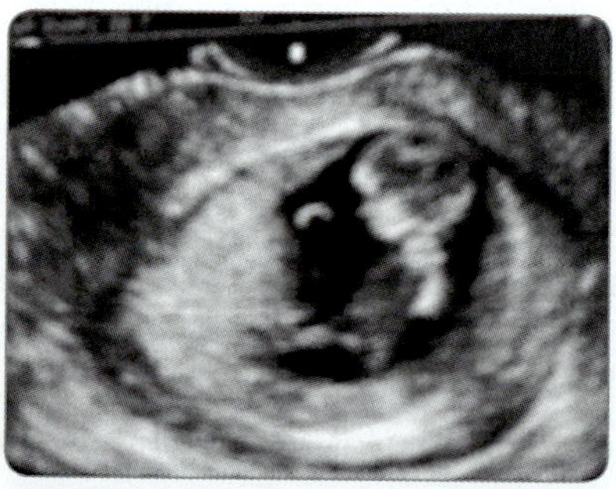

Fig. 2: Ultrasonography of early pregnancy

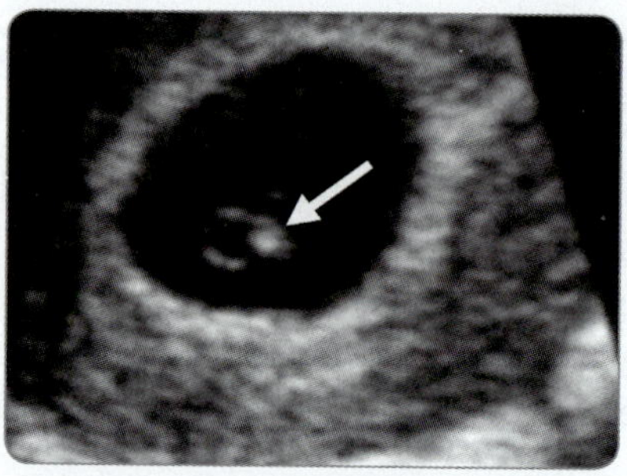

Fig. 3: Gestational sac of early pregnancy with yolk sac (arrow)

pregnancy is of help. With this method implanted gestational sac has been identified as early as at four weeks menstrual age.

Assessment of Gestational Age

In first trimester, gestational age is determined by the volume of the sac, presence of fetal echo complex, fetal heart movements, crown-rump length and even fetal movement.

Presence of yolk sac confirms intrauterine pregnancy. An intrauterine gestational sac can be seen by 6th week by transabdominal sonography (TAS) and from 5th week by transvaginal sonography (TVS). At this time the volume of the gestational sac is 1 mL and at 13th week of pregnancy it is 100 mL; the shape is round. By seventh week the fetal echo is clearly visible. Then it is possible to measure the crown-rump length. Fetal heart movement is also visible along with fetal body movement. Cardiac activity is usually seen with the appearance of the embryo by 5 to 5½ weeks by TVS and 6 to 6½ weeks by TAS. Crown-rump length can be used to determine gestational age upto 12th week only, after that it is less accurate. Several graphs are available for this purpose.

Bleeding in Early Pregnancy

Bleeding per vaginum in early weeks of pregnancy is a common complication. Sometimes it is very difficult for the attending doctor to determine whether the

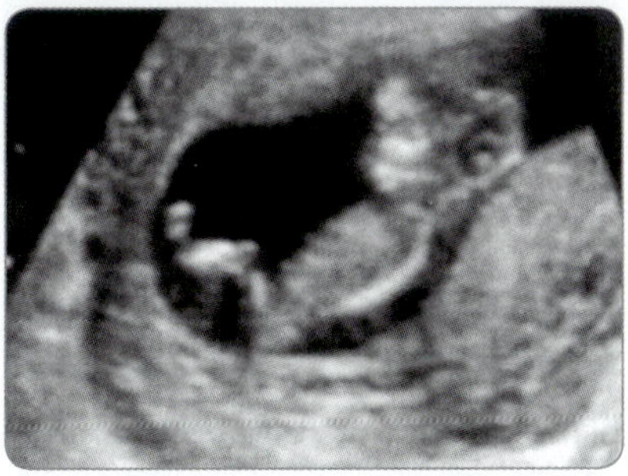

Fig. 4: Ultrasonography of 12 weeks of pregnancy

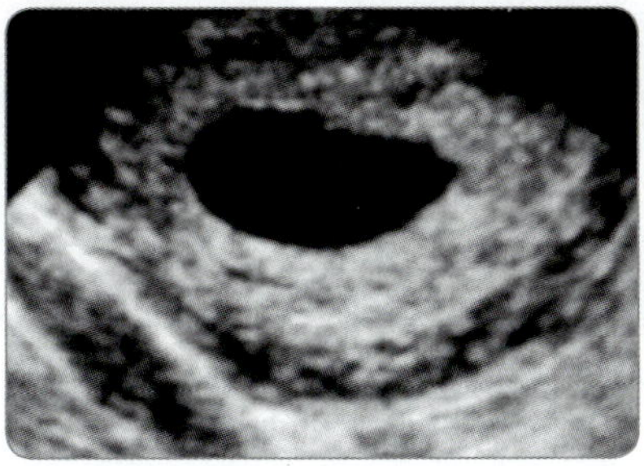

Fig. 5: Ultrasonography of anembryonic sac

pregnancy is intact or is going to be aborted. In such situation ultrasonographic examination of the gestational sac is very helpful. In abortion the gestational sac is poorly outlined or deformed. After 8 weeks of pregnancy absence of fetal echo and fetal heart movement are abnormal signs. When abortion is complete the uterus is empty and smaller than the period of gestation.

Another important cause of early pregnancy bleeding is vesicular mole or hydatidiform mole. Ultrasonography can diagnose vesicular mole accurately (Fig. 6).

The typical "snow storm" pattern may not be visualized in all the cases.

Ectopic Pregnancy

Ectopic pregnancy is a condition where ultrasonographic help is sought frequently. In this condition the bulky uterus is empty, cystic or semicystic lesion is present in one adnexa and free fluid in the pouch of Douglus (Fig. 7).

In Second and Third Trimester

In second and third trimester the fetus in utero can be studied in great detail. Information regarding the head, spine, the abdomen, thorax and limbs are obtained along with the position of the placenta and amount of liquor amnii.

During this period of gestation the important indications of ultrasonography are:

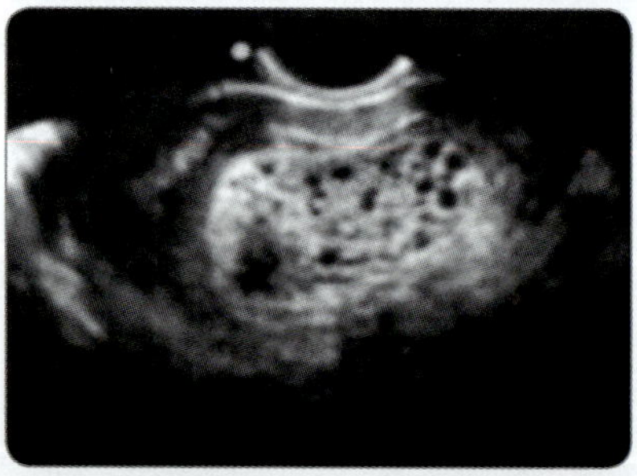

Fig. 6: Ultrasonography of hydatidiform mole (Note the typical "snow storm" appearance)

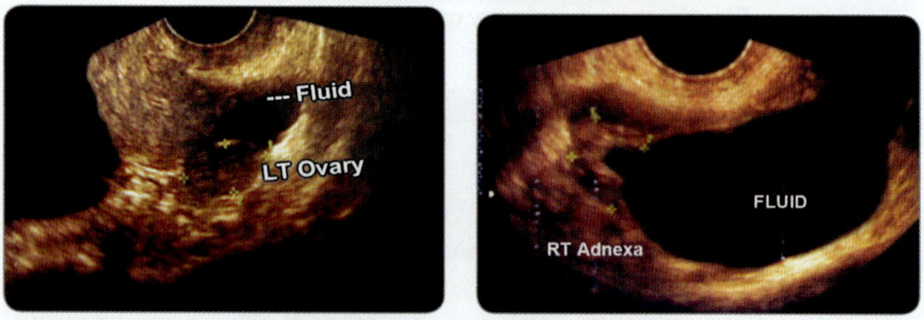

Fig. 7: Ultrasonography of disturbed ectopic pregnancy (Note collection of blood in right adnexa)

- To determine the gestational age
- To diagnose intrauterine growth restriction
- To detect congenital anomalies of the fetus
- To find out the cause of bleeding per vaginum
- In certain situations to guide amniocentesis
- Diagnosis of intrauterine fetal death
- Localization of placenta.

Estimation of Gestational Age

In second and third trimester gestational age is estimated by biparietal diameter (BPD), femur length, head circumference and binocular distance. By 13–14 weeks biparietal diameter can be measured. From 14th week to 30th week the BPD is an almost accurate method to determine gestational age. So for determination of the gestational age, BPD measurement is obtained around 14–20 weeks. Sometimes a second measurement is needed after about 2 weeks of the first scanning. During this period intrauterine growth restriction does not effect the measurement. Sometimes the second measurement is taken around 28–30 weeks. It is prudent to take measurement of two different fetal parameters to avoid error in estimation.

Intrauterine Growth Restriction

The final diagnosis of intrauterine growth restriction (IUGR) can be made only after delivery of the baby, where the birth weight is less than 10th percentile for the corresponding gestational age. Clinical diagnosis of the condition is not easy. Serial ultrasonographic measurements of diferent fetal parameters can give an accurate diagnosis of IUGR. For this purpose BPD, length of the femur, head circumference, abdominal circumference are essential. Along with these measurements assessment of amount of liquor amnii is important as oligohydramnios usually accompanies fetal growth restriction. If the pocket of amniotic fluid is less than 1 cm, olygohydramnios is diagnosed. Ideally the first USG should be done before 20 weeks of gestation, the second at 28th week and then at 34–36 weeks. Fetal weight is also estimated from these parameters.

Detection of Congenital Anomalies

Ultrasonography plays an important role in antenatal diagnosis of different congenital malformation of the fetus. The anomalies which can be detected by ultrasound are central nervous system anomalies like anencephalus, hydrocephalus, microcephalus, spina bifida; gastrointestinal anomalies like omphalocele, duodenal atresia, diaphragmatic hernia, fetal ascites; in excretory system, renal dysplasia, multiple polycystic kidney, renal agenesis, bladder neck obstruction; congenital cardiac anomalies and achondroplasia, etc. In high-risk cases anomaly scan should be performed before 20 weeks of pregnancy so that, if needed pregnancy can be terminated safely. Nowadays a routine first scan is advised at 10–11 weeks of gestation to detect congenital abnormality.

Bleeding in Late Pregnancy

One major cause of late pregnancy bleeding is low lying placenta. With the help of ultrasonography placenta previa can be diagnosed almost accurately.

Intrauterine Fetal Death

Clinical diagnosis of intrauterine fetal death is not difficult, but sometimes ultasonography is helpful. Besides distortion of fetal skull, over-riding of skull bones are important signs. However, absence of visible heart beat is the most reliable sign of fetal death.

❐ CERVICAL INCOMPETENCE

Cervical incompetence is an important cause of mid-trimester abortion. Ultrasonographic examination of cervix is performed to evaluate the integrity of the cervix. Length of the cervix, width of the cervical canal and funelling of the upper cervical canal are important parameters. Normal cervical length during pregnancy is 2.5 to 6 cm and cervix remains closed. In incompetent cervix the length is less than 2.5 cm, width of the internal os is more than 15 mm in second trimester or more than 8 mm in third trimester, funelling of cervix more than 2 cm. TVS is of more advantage than AVS to detect cervical incompetence.

Other conditions where ultrasonography is of help are hydramnios, and multiple pregnancy. When hydramnios is diagnosed clinically ultrasonography is indicated to exclude any congenital fetal anomaly. Similarity in multiple pregnancy also besides identifying multiple fetuses care is taken to exclude fetal anomaly and low lying placenta. In cases with extrapelvic lump USG is used to determine the nature of the lump, namely ovarian tumor and uterine fibroid. Nowadays introduction of Doppler velocimetry in ultrasound technology has facilitated the study of maternal and fetal circulatory functions. With this advanced technique placental blood flow can be studied along with blood flow through umbilical artery and through the major arteries of the fetus. Hence, uteroplacental blood flow and fetal cardiac activities can be studied and placental insufficiency can be diagnosed early. Another method to assess fetal well-being by ultrasound is fetal biophysical profile. In this procedure different fetal activities and amount of liquor amnii are assessed and fetal condition is evaluated.

Ultrasonography is a safe method. Till date no confirmed biological effect on the mother or on the developing fetus has been reported. But still its use should be judicious and a patient should be subjected to ultrasonographic examination only when genuinely indicated.

❐ USG IN GYNECOLOGY

Determination of Pelvic Mass

The origin, size and consistency of a pelvic mass can be evaluated. Differentiation of uterine fibromyoma, ovarian tumor, tubo-ovarian mass, endometrioma can be made. In case of fibromyoma of uterus its number, exact location and size can be determined before operation is planned.

Endometrial Pathology

Presence of endometrial hyperplasia, polyp or retained product of conception can be detected (Fig. 8). TVS is more helpful than abdominal sonography. Unexplained irregular bleeding or post-menopausal bleeding should be evaluated by transvaginal sonography.

Pelvic Malignancy

A malignant ovarian tumor may be of increased size, partly solid and partly cystic. The morphologic characteristics of malignant tumor are heterogeneous texture, thick septa with papillary vegetation.

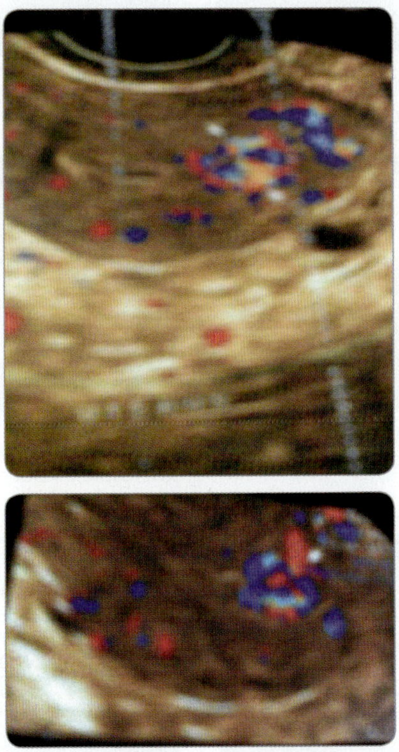

Fig. 8: Ultrasonography (Doppler) of uterus shows retained product inside

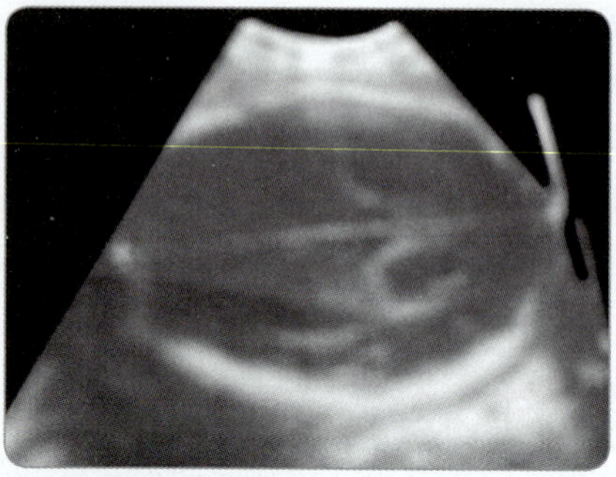

Fig. 9: Fetal biparietal diameter

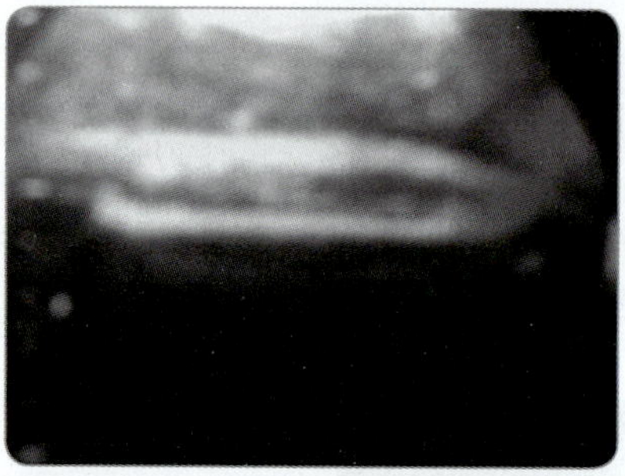

Fig. 10: Ultrasonography of near term pregnancy showing the femur

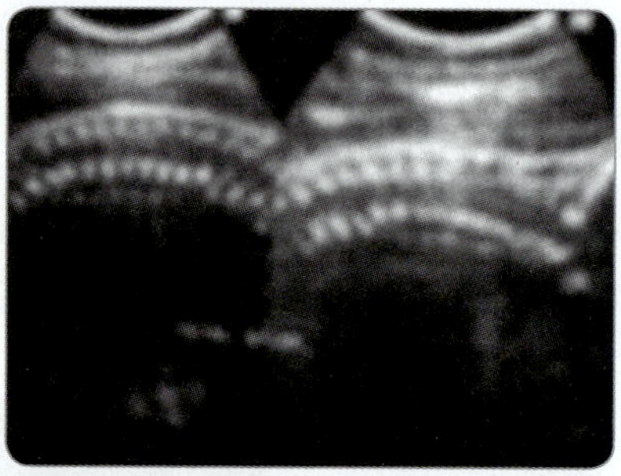

Fig. 11: Ultrasonography of term pregnancy showing fetal spine

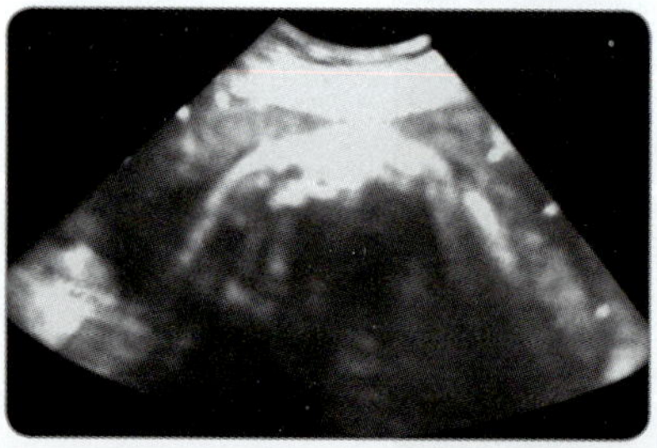

Fig. 12: Ultrasonography of term pregnancy shows umbilical cord around the fetal neck

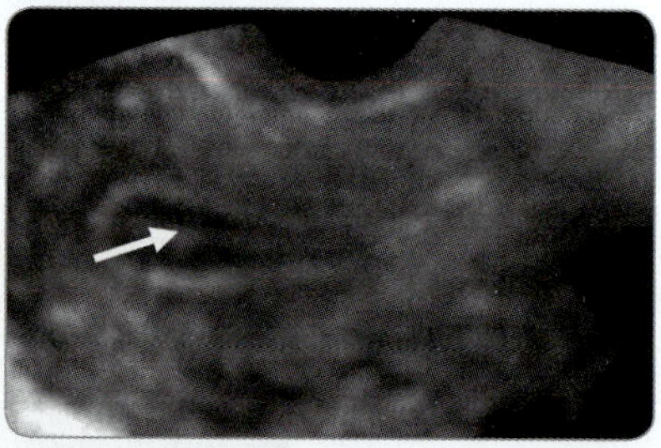

Fig. 13: Ultrasonography of uterus shows the triple line of endometrium (arrow)

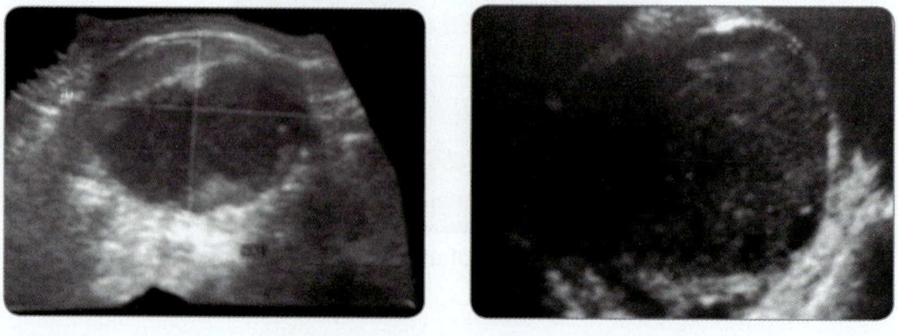

Fig. 14: Chocolate cyst of ovary

Blood flow pattern in a tumor can be studied by color Doppler imaging and its abnormality gives significant clue to the nature of the tumor. Additional findings of malignancy are neovascularity, low impedance, etc.

In Infertility

Ultrasonography evaluation plays an important role in initial evaluation of the patient. Other indications are:

- Folliculometry–Serial measurement of ovarian follicular size and endometrial thickness are carried out to detect ovulation. Ovulation is detected by appearance of internal echos, diminished size of the follicle and presence of free fluid in pouch of Douglas.
- Oocyte retrieval in IVF is done under ultrasound guidance.

Sonohysterography

Saline solution is instilled inside the uterine cavity and when studied by TVS submucous fibromyoma, endometrial polyp can be diagnosed easily.

Ultrasonography can be used to determine tubal patency. Normal saline is pushed inside the uterine cavity passing a catheter through the cervix. Ultrasound can follow the flow of fluid through the tubes. Patency is confirmed by appearance of fluid in pouch of Douglas. This is called sonosalpingography.

Another indication is to locate a missed IUCD, whether it is inside or outside the uterine cavity (Fig. 16).

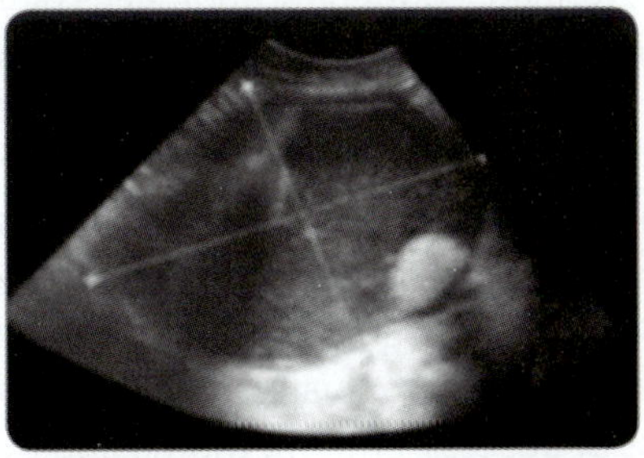

Fig. 15: Dermoid cyst of ovary

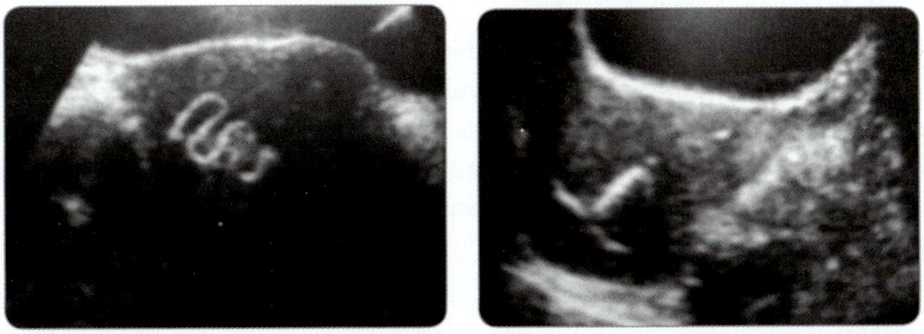

Fig. 16: Intrauterine contraceptive devices seen inside the uterine cavity

Ultrasonography is helpful to carry out some procedures, as aspiration of chocolate cyst, aspiration of tubo-ovarian abscess and to take biopsy. In IVF clinic ultrasonographic assisted ovum retrieval is done.

❐ COMPUTED TOMOGRAPHY

CT scan provides multiple cross-sectional images of the part of the body at short distance. In gynecology CT scan helps to evaluate pelvic mass particularly in staging of malignant conditions.

Cervical Carcinoma

CT scan is indicated in poorly differentiated, bulky tumor mass. It can detect metastatic lymph nodes in pelvis and extension of the lesion to the pelvic wall. It can diagnose hydroureter, hydronephrosis or bowel involvement by the lesion. Thereby can eliminate the need of intravenous urography or barium enema.

CT scan is not used in obstetrics, due to irradiation.

❐ MAGNETIC RESONANCE IMAGING

MRI also provides cross-sectional images of the body. MRI is indicated only when USG diagnosis is inadequate or for staging of carcinoma. It gives excellent soft tissue detail of pelvic organs. No doubt it is superior to USG or CT scan but it is more expensive.

MRI can clearly differentiate congenital anomalies of uterus. Fibromyoma of uterus are better diagnosed with details. It is indicated in cases of endometrial carcinoma where it can clearly demonstrate myometrial involvement of the disease.

In carcinoma cervix it is used to know accurately, the parametrial invasion by the carcinoma. Metastasis to urinary bladder and rectum can be demonstrated.

MRI is superior to CT in detecting lymph gland metastasis in any pelvic malignancy. It can also be used to evaluate origin and nature of any pelvic mass like tubo-ovarian mass or abscess, endometrioma and ovarian tumor.

❐ IN OBSTETRICS

The role of MRI is not well-established in the field of obstetrics. No irradiation is used in MRI but still its possible adverse effects on unborn fetus is not fully evaluated. In obstetrics USG is the better option though MRI can provide clear information about fetal anomaly, intrauterine fetal death, site of placentation and placental pathology. USG is easier and cheaper procedure and undoubtedly the method of choice.

Index

Page numbers followed by *f* refer to figure.

C

T

U